Praise for *Move Into Life: NeuroMove*

D0455898

"When I interviewed Anat and later rea and stunned. Anat has a remarkably so of how the brain changes IN PRACTICE; a total connection with the enormous potential of the brain; A detailed and practical understanding of how to recruit learning capabilities and a framework she has carefully constructed over decades that allows her gift to be TAUGHT to trainees."

— Martha Herbert, M.D. Harvard Medical School, MGH, ABM practitioner, author of *The Autism Revolution*

"Essential reading for anyone seeking to enhance their physical and mental performance and vitality. Based on sound science, the Nine Essentials of the Anat Baniel Method are not only easy to incorporate into daily life, they are pleasurable, highly effective, and invigorating."

— Daniel Graupe, PhD, University of Illinois, Chicago, Illinois

"*Move into Life* is a brilliant and original approach to bringing about rapid change and enhanced vitality. This program gives you access to the limitless energy and vibrancy that are at the heart of a happy and satisfying life."

—Marci Shimoff, New York Times bestselling author of *Happy for No Reason*

"Anat Baniel is a pioneer. As someone lucky enough to have experienced this work first hand I'll always keep this book in my reference library. This is information that changes the way you think about body mechanics. We are holographic beings. The thigh bone is connected to the foot bone is connected to the toe bone. Give this book to your physical therapist, your rehab facility administrator and your orthopedic surgeon!"

—Allison Peacock, reader review, Amazon.com

"Anat's ideas are simple: pay attention while you move, move slowly, use less force, do whatever you are doing in new ways, do new things, be flexible, enthusiastic, and above all, be aware of what you are feeling. I first heard of Anat's work two years ago. And, at the age of 65, I signed up for her basic training. It is difficult to describe transformational changes and make them believable. I don't just feel a little younger. I have learned to better use my body. I walk firmly over my skeleton, upright, with an energy unknown to me, at least in my adult life. I easily keep up with my grandchildren."

— Elizabeth Elgin, reader review, Amazon.com

"I found this book just in time! I love my family, but I was tired of the routine, the laundry, the dishes. You get it. I was walking around half-attentive to everything because I was always weary and, frankly, bored. The simple, yet profound ideas in *Move Into Life* have transformed me and my life. I have energy to enjoy my family and have been inspired to start a new, exciting career. I'm thrilled and I am sharing this book with everyone in my life. Strong recommendation! Buy this and then REALLY DO THE EXERCISES! Do not skip them! It's worth every moment."

—Meta L. McDaniel, reader review, Amazon.com

"For 30 years, through mastery, pure genius, Baniel has created transformational changes within the brains, minds and bodies of the children and adults she has worked with. Through her book, she offers readers accessible and pleasurable strategies and techniques to create transformational changes in their own brains as they move through the course of their daily lives. In learning to 'wake up' our own brain, we discover how to become more productive, fulfilled and youthful human beings. Reading this book will turn on your own "Learning Switch," creating a more vital and healthful present and future... creates a new and expansive vision for every reader."

—Abigail Natenshon, MA, LCSW, GCFP, author of *When Your Child Has an Eating Disorder: A Step-by-Step Workbook for Parents and Other Caregivers*

Other works by Anat Baniel

- *Kids Beyond Limits: The Anat Baniel Method for Awakening the Brain and Transforming the Life of Your Special Needs Child* (Paperback and ebook)
- *NeuroMovement® for Whole Body Fitness (Video)*
- *NeuroMovement® for Better Balance (Video)*
- *NeuroMovement® for Healthy Dynamic Sitting (Video)*
- *NeuroMovement® for Healthy Breathing (Video)*
- *NeuroMovement® for Healthy Backs (Video)*
- *NeuroMovement® for Healthy Necks and Shoulders (Video)*
- *NeuroMovement® for Healthy Backs, Scoliosis & Pain Relief (Video)*
- *NeuroMovement® for Healthy Backs (Audio)*
- *NeuroMovement® for Healthy Necks (Audio)*
- *NeuroMovement® for Healthy Joints (Audio)*
- *NeuroMovement® for Children with Special Needs 2-Day Workshop (Video)*

Coming Soon

- *NeuroMovement® for Vitality, Anti-Aging and Well-Being 5-Day Workshop (Video)*
- *NeuroMovement® for Parent and Child with Special Needs 5-Day Workshop (Video)*

Anat Baniel Method Center

NeuroMovement for Whole Brain and Body Fitness

MOVE INTO LIFE

NeuroMovement®
for Lifelong Vitality

Anat Baniel

Illustrations by David Gerstein

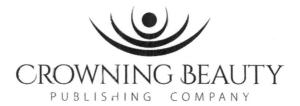

CROWNING BEAUTY
PUBLISHING COMPANY

The stories in this book are true. Names, circumstances, and identifying characteristics of the participants have been changed to protect their anonymity and to respect client confidentiality.

For information regarding this book and other media by this author, contact: Crowning Beauty Publishing Company, 4330 Redwood Highway, Suite 350, San Rafael, CA 94903. Telephone 800-386-1441.

For further information regarding the work described herein, visit: www.AnatBanielMethod.com

The terms Anat Baniel Method®, NeuroMovement®, and The Nine Essentials® are the property of Anat Baniel.

Illustrations by David Gerstein.

Cover art by Clifford Schinkel.

ISBN-13: 978-1519438881
ISBN-10: 1519438885

To my parents, Malka and Avram Baniel,
who knew that I could.

To my beloved teacher, mentor, and friend Moshe Feldenkrais,
who showed me the way.

There are only two ways to live your life. One is as though nothing is a miracle, the other is as though everything is a miracle.

—ALBERT EINSTEIN

Contents

FOREWORD XI

INTRODUCTION I

VITALITY AND YOUTHFULNESS 5

THE NINE ESSENTIALS

ONE   MOVEMENT WITH ATTENTION—
        WAKE UP TO LIFE 23

TWO   THE LEARNING SWITCH—
        BRING IN THE NEW 48

THREE   SUBTLETY—EXPERIENCE THE POWER
        OF GENTLENESS 81

FOUR   VARIATION—ENJOY ABUNDANT
        POSSIBILITIES 106

FIVE   SLOW—LUXURIATE IN THE RICHNESS
        OF FEELING 34

SIX   ENTHUSIASM—TURN THE SMALL
        INTO THE GREAT 156

SEVEN   FLEXIBLE GOALS—MAKE THE
         IMPOSSIBLE POSSIBLE 182

EIGHT   IMAGINATION AND DREAMS—CREATE
         YOUR LIFE 206

NINE   AWARENESS—THRIVE WITH TRUE
         KNOWLEDGE 234

         MOVE INTO LIFE 253

Notes 263
Bibliography 291
Acknowledgments 295
Index 299
About Anat Baniel 305
Anat Baniel Method Center 308

MOVE INTO LIFE

NeuroMovement®
for Lifelong Vitality

Foreword

Advances in neuroscience have radically changed how we think about the brain, and this is good news for any of us looking forward to enjoying our later years. Rather than seeing the brain as an organ that matures over the first twenty years of our lives and then withers away with the years, scientists now view the human brain as constantly changing. Dendrites, those thousands of tentacle-like receptors that extend from the ends of most of the nerve cells in your brain, can rapidly grow and retreat in periods of a couple weeks. These neuronal changes can even occur in a matter of minutes regardless of one's age! Akira Yoshii, a brain researcher at MIT, states that: "The development of particular neurological connections or skills does not occur gradually over time. Instead, such changes tend to occur suddenly, appearing in short intervals after robust stimulation. It is as if there is a single important trigger and then a functional circuit rapidly comes online."

The Nobel laureate Eric Kendel proved that neurons never stop learning. He demonstrated that if you alter the environmental stimulus, the internal function of our nerve cells will change, causing them to grow new extensions, called axons, capable of communicating new and different information to other parts of our brains. Every change in our environment, whether internal and external, will cause a rearrangement of neuronal activity and growth. In fact, every neuron in our brain has its own "mind," capable of deciding whether to send a signal or not, and how strong a signal to send once it makes that decision. Think about that for a moment: you have 80 billion tiny minds living inside your brain, and they cooperate as well as the finest symphony in the world.

Scientists used to believe that our neurons deteriorated with age, but the newest research shows that we can "exercise" the brain in the same way we exercise our bodies. Instead of weights, we can use our thoughts to eliminate physical and mental stress. We can strengthen our social awareness circuits to feel more empathy for others and self-love for ourselves, and we can weaken the neural connections that cause us to become overly anxious or depressed. As I have stated in my own books, including *Words Can Change Your Brain*, our research demonstrates that even something as subtle as the words we choose to use can help us to maintain a healthy structural balance in our brains. This brings me to Anat Baniel's work.

Over 30 years ago, the author of *Move Into Life* had begun to observe in her clients how the brain responds to certain conditions, generating information in the brain, and how the brain's new organization of that information was often experienced as increased vitality. Clients recovering from accidents or other health problems — as well as those who came to her seeking relief from aches, pains, and limitations ordinarily associated with aging — noticed considerable improvement. They moved with greater ease and strength, their thinking was clearer, they felt stronger and more confident, and their sense of well-being greatly improved. They were exercising their brains, building better connections that could transform their lives. transform their lives. That's the power of neuroplasticity, and Anat understood how to help her students and clients achieve these remarkable transformations.

Anat created "Nine Essentials" that I consider to be brilliant. For example, her principle of moving slowly to create greater awareness has now been documented by neuroscience. She brings in the importance of playfulness and imagination, two of the most important but often overlooked strategies for maintaining neurological health. Her Nine Essentials® are the conditions the brain needs to bring about potent positive change. *Move Into Life* is a book that I think everyone should read and use, and I only wish that her Nine Essentials® were taught to every child in every school throughout the world. We need to exercise the brain, and there are too few people teaching us how we can move our bodies in ways that bring greater clarity of our thinking.

Thanks to Anat's lifelong interest in the human brain and her commitment to teaching others these remarkable techniques, everyone can now gain immediate access to building a better brain. How wonderful it is to have a book filled with clear and simple instructions for improving our functioning and vitality for many years to come.

—Mark Robert Waldman, executive MBA Faculty, Loyola Marymount University. His book *Words Can Change Your Brain* is a "New York Times" bestseller.

Introduction

Since the publication of the first edition of *Move Into Life* I coined the term NeuroMovement® to describe not only the Anat Baniel Method®, but the remarkable opportunity we have as adults to continuously improve our lives, to be healthier, smarter, stronger and happier, to live longer and make our additional years fulfilling and productive.

When I began this work, over 30 years ago, there was little in the scientific literature to support what I observed nearly every day in my work, through the improvements in my students' lives and in what these changes were revealing to me about the brain.

During those early years, and in spite of evidence that I was seeing to the contrary, science generally presumed that our vitality and ability to learn peaks in our early twenties. From then on, the only way was down, and there was little we could do about it. It was believed that our brains stop growing and evolving after the first few years of life and can only change for the worse after that.

More recently, much has been published in the field of brain research known as brain plasticity, or simply, neuroplasticity, which validates what I had been observing in my work—that in fact our brains are able to evolve and change throughout our lives. This has been demonstrated on cellular levels as well as in *cortical remapping*, wherein the growth of new neural pathways becomes possible.

It was therefore deeply gratifying for me when Michael Merzenich, PhD, Professor Emeritus at University of California in San Francisco, and one of the foremost pioneers in this new science of the brain, wrote the following in his foreword to my second book, *Kids Beyond Limits*: "I have spent much of my own scientific career trying to understand how we can harness our capacity for brain remodeling for the benefit of children and adults. From several decades of research...we scientists have defined the 'rules' governing brain plasticity in neurological terms. Anat Baniel, working in parallel along a completely different path has defined almost exactly the same rules...and interprets them here in practical and understandable human terms, in ways that should contribute richly to your life."

I witness the creative potentials of the human brain every day in my work. Whether teaching a trauma victim to trust again, or an athlete to achieve his personal best, or a small child with serious neurological challenges to gain fuller use of her body and mind, or helping a man or woman of any age gain physical, mental, and emotional flexibility and strength, it is always through the miracles of the brain's plasticity that I see their vitality emerge. It is through NeuroMovement and the Nine Essentials, which I describe in this book, that we are able to intentionally facilitate the brain's innate abilities to change and repair itself.

What today is known as The Anat Baniel Method, which incorporates NeuroMovement and The Nine Essentials, evolved from my background in clinical psychology, my passion for the sciences, dance, the work of Dr. Moshe Feldenkrais—a physicist and pioneer in the mind-body field—and a thriving practice that has spanned more than three decades, working with thousands of people from five days old to ninety years of age; from high-performance athletes, business people, scientists, and musicians to people worn down by daily stress or aches and pains, to those seeking greater freedom, fulfillment, and joy in their life.

Many of my students, especially in the earlier years of my career, came to me after being told by their doctors, therapists, teachers, and others what was *not possible* for them. Often this was like a verdict from on high telling them they would just have to accept their present limitations and learn to live with them. I knew that if I could somehow find a way to communicate with their brains, and get their brains to resume growing, creating, and inventing new solutions, then the possibilities would be endless and often surprising.

The recent research in neuroplasticity clearly demonstrates that our brains can continue to grow, develop, and change throughout life. What I didn't expect was that each time I worked with my students, their vitality emerged and grew. It has been my privilege and ongoing delight to observe my students, during private sessions, workshops, and training programs, become stronger and freer in body, mind, emotion, and spirit, shedding limitations, becoming more energetic, their thinking getting clearer and more creative as they live their lives more fully.

The consistency of the results my students have gotten from this work has led me to search, and eventually define, key requirements— the Nine Essentials—for our brains to wake up, grow beyond past limitation, and thrive, rewarding us with greater flexibility in body and mind, with enhanced strength, intelligence, well-being, and ability to relate to others. Once defined, anyone can benefit from the Nine Essentials.

In *Move Into Life* you will learn what these Nine Es-sentials are, what and how you can easily apply them in your daily life. These essentials are not a list of what you should or should not do. They are the underpinnings of NeuroMovement, the conditions you can provide for a better working brain in whatever you do, and for you to thrive. The essentials are easy to grasp, almost obvious, once you learn what they are. For each essential there is a vitality quotient questionnaire that lets you know how well you are doing with that essential. You can begin applying the essentials as you read about them and begin experiencing changes right away.

This book will help you discover what is possible for you. You don't need to have a problem or be experiencing limitation to obtain great benefit from this method. Life's inevitable stresses and challenges cause wear and tear on everyone's vitality. If you feel stuck, bored, low on energy, or resigned or hopeless in any area of your life, or if you have an injury or illness, your brain needs extra help to move you out of your rut and into life. Through NeuroMovement and the Nine Essentials your brain can move to higher levels of functioning and infuse you with greater delight, energy, creativity, and success. My hope is for you to pick up this book, read it, and begin applying the essentials right away. My certainty is that when you do, your life will become richer, more interesting and fulfilling, and you will be rewarded with the vitality and joy that you seek.

Vitality and Youthfulness

You are never too old to become younger!

—Mae West

While flying home from teaching a NeuroMovement® training in Chicago, it suddenly dawned on me that each time a student or client of mine improved, she or he radiated vitality. Their faces relaxed and their skin color became more vibrant. Their eyes brightened. Their voices became more enthusiastic and melodious. They stood taller and with greater ease. They exuded a sense of peacefulness and quiet attentiveness. They moved with greater grace, energy, flexibility, and confidence. When I am able to observe my students over several hours or days, as is often the case in my longer seminars, I notice their thinking becomes clearer and their ability to express themselves sharper. They laugh more and become lighter in spirit—they get my jokes! They exhibit radiant beauty that comes from a place deep within them and is reflected in every part of their demeanor.

At the time of this realization, I had been working with a great variety of people, men and women from all walks of life, all ages and conditions. I saw people such as the sixty-year-old executive recovering from a stroke, the thirty-year-old mother recovering from a difficult childbirth, and the forty-year-old sales representative wanting to improve his golf game. I even worked with students from the university who were in perfect health but were searching for ways to improve their academic performance and creative capacities. Many were referred to me by a friend or spouse who had benefited from NeuroMovement; their lives had been going fine, but the workshops opened up new possibilities for them. There were also world-class musicians, dancers, and athletes searching for ways to improve their performance. In addition, I had been doing a great deal with infants and children with developmental problems, which had informed me so much about what we adults need in order to thrive. Over the years, I have helped thousands of people move beyond their present limitations, whether those limitations were intellectual, emotional, physical, or even the result of genetics.

No matter who they were or why they came, all who opened their minds to this work had one thing in common—they radiated *vitality*.

Reclaim Your Vitality

Whether you have experienced vitality for brief or extended periods of time, it is not something you easily forget. You might remember falling in love and feeling filled with energy, light on your feet, and hopeful about the future. Or perhaps you remember getting your dream job and then bursting with creative new ideas. If you play tennis or golf, or some other sport, you may have had the experience, many times over, of exceeding your personal best and feeling flooded with energy, ready to perform at higher and higher levels. You might recall the deep vitality you felt while making love passionately, or the thrill and empowerment you experienced when you found a new way to increase your income or make a career change. Vitality is something we all know, regardless of our activities and interests. If nothing else, we have all experienced vitality in our childhoods, during the period of our steepest learning curves when our brains were constantly generating new information, forming new patterns, and creating new possibilities in our lives.

For a moment, think about your life in the first hours following your birth. Reflect on how much you have grown and evolved to be where you are today. In those early hours in your mother's arms, you responded to touch, sound, light, movement, and the comfort or discomfort of your body, but you had yet to develop anything resembling voluntary action. You could initiate very little, except perhaps to follow a movement with your eyes, suckle, or cry. For many months, even years, your growth seemed to take care of itself. While you were dependent on others to provide emotional, physical, and mental support, the curve of your development was extraordinarily steep, like a race up a mountain path.

During this time, you were bursting at the seams with energy, curiosity, and spontaneous creativity—and with it came the fire of vitality that made so much of your experience exhilarating. The vitality you experienced in those early years was directly connected to the fact that behind the scenes your brain was growing new connections and patterns at the staggering rate of 1.8 million connections per second. Each new set of patterns provided you with new possibilities for movement, feeling, thought, and action. Nearly every day, you developed new capacities and discovered new things. Life was exhilarating. What happened between then and now to diminish this vitality?

Very simply, when we get to a certain level of development, most of us begin to coast. We stop providing our brains with what they need in order to continue to grow and create new possibilities for us. Our brains either slow way down or stop forming new connections altogether; as a result, we begin repeating the same patterns over and over again. Eventually, with no significant change, our lives become habitual, and we begin to deteriorate in the ways we think, move, and feel.

As adults, we find ways of thinking and doing that work for us, ways that are usually productive, efficient, and practical. Then we repeat those patterns again and again. After all, we can't reinvent the wheel every time we get up in the morning or drive to work or do routine tasks our jobs require. We'd never get through the day without having efficient routines and habits we can rely on. The downside is that we can become like automatons running the same old circuits day after day. ways that are usually productive, efficient, and practical. Then we repeat those patterns again and again. After all, we can't reinvent the wheel every time we get up in the morning or drive to work or do routine tasks our jobs require. We'd never get through the day without having efficient routines and habits we can rely on. The downside is that we can become like automatons running the same old circuits day after day.

But part of our true nature is to go beyond persistent habit and routine. Our brains thrive when creating new information, and this is what we require to feel alive and enthusiastic—vitally engaged in our lives. When we don't provide our brains with what they need in order to create and thrive, we begin to feel lethargic and inflexible. We get aches and pains, and we become less and less responsive to people and events around us. The more this occurs, the more new information seems like a distraction or even a threat to us. We become physically and mentally dull, increasingly unreceptive to anything that seems new or different.

Is it possible to reignite our vitality at will, regardless of our age, physical symptoms, or station in life? The answer is *yes*! You can have the high levels of vitality you long for, and you can recreate it throughout your life. Our brains have an innate capacity to keep discovering and inventing new ways of acting and thinking. They are most vibrant and alive when called upon to differentiate, that is, to recognize finer and finer distinctions and make increasingly finer choices, to form new patterns and reach higher levels of complexity, skill, comfort, strength, and heightened levels of performance in everything we do.

Through NeuroMovement and the Nine Essentials, you'll learn about what your brain needs to thrive. You will have the opportunity to experience simple, subtle body movements and mental exercises that satisfy those needs and thus awaken your vitality. You'll also discover why and how these methods work, based on research and my experience over the past thirty years. And you'll find that the practical applications of these methods are so intuitive that you'll find it easy to integrate them into all areas of your everyday life.

Over and over again, I see people come to life who have felt dead and torpid, trapped by restricting circumstances, sometimes for many years. I have seen people who have suffered the energy-blunting experience of chronic pain, experienced the disappointment of a stunted life based on rigid and limiting beliefs, or deadened by a life of routine, reawaken their brains and regain the vitality that makes life worth living. They often describe their experience with phrases such as: "I feel twenty years younger!" or "I feel like a kid again!" or "I have never felt better in my life!" or "I didn't know this was possible" or "Now I know I can follow my dream." They discover their capacity to enjoy greater freedom, flexibility, and strength, with enormous bursts of energy and joy.

EXERCISE 1   TRANSFORMATION THROUGH WHAT YOU DON'T YET KNOW

Most of us have experienced the feeling that "I've tried everything and nothing works." This usually comes while struggling with a difficult situation and settling on the belief, at least for the moment, that what you wanted to happen is impossible. What often proves to be true is not that you had really *tried everything*, but that you had believed in your own limitations; that is, you'd believed in the limited knowledge you had at that moment. New solutions and new possibilities await us in what we don't yet know, or in what hasn't yet evolved.

Think of a time when you felt stuck and then, with new knowledge, created a solution that changed everything for the better. This might have been in a relationship challenge, a work-related problem, your sexuality, your health, or in a recreational activity. Let this be your reminder that there is always something beyond what you presently know; you need not limit yourself to your present knowledge. Dare to believe in what may seem impossible.

There's a wonderful exchange between Alice and the White Queen in Lewis Carroll's *Through the Looking-Glass*. When Alice complains that she can't believe impossible things, the Queen replies: "I daresay you haven't had much practice . . . When I was your age I always did it for half-an-hour a day. Why, sometimes I believed as many as six impossible things before breakfast."

EXERCISE 2   THE TRANSFORMATIONAL POWER OF KNOWLEDGE

Take a few moments and create a list of at least one time when you were sure something was impossible for you to have or accomplish and that later on, with new knowledge, became possible. Then continue adding to this list every day. It can be from any aspect of your life: physical, emotional, mental, relationship, faith, work, financial, or recreational activity. It can be a recent experience, or something you experienced a long time ago. Practice this skill until you become an expert in knowing that with additional knowledge, you can move beyond what you believe to be impossible.

TRANSFORMATION FOR A BETTER LIFE

Over the years, I have experienced the joy of working with thousands of people—teachers, accountants, homemakers, truck drivers, lawyers, grandmothers, professors, secretaries, and others. Many faces come to mind as examples of the transformational process people experience as they move beyond what they once perceived as personal limitations, ultimately achieving capacities they had only dreamed were possible. Madison's story is particularly powerful. On the surface, her situation shows how pain—be it physical or mental—can compromise our lives, making it difficult, or impossible, to do even that which we love. It was pain that motivated her to seek help, but it doesn't have to be. Madison's story speaks to anyone wanting to enjoy greater vitality and joy.

When Madison walked into a crowded room, people sat up and took notice, captivated by her exceptional air of self-confidence and professionalism. At forty-two, she appeared ten years younger— slender, brunette, five-foot-nine, and smartly dressed. A successful businesswoman, she was president of her own consulting firm, coaching executives in key organizations. Happily married to a San Francisco attorney, her life seemed ideal.

I first met Madison when she enrolled in my workshop at the Anat Baniel Method Center in San Rafael, California. I started out this workshop by having the participants form a large circle, then asking them to introduce themselves and say what they wished to accomplish in the class. The circle that day consisted of several professional people, including a musician from a symphony orchestra, a couple of school teachers, a psychotherapist, and a surgeon. There were housewives, retired men and women, and a college girl who was studying biology. All had their own reasons for coming to the workshop, ranging from the retired doctor recovering from depression to the young father grappling with panic attacks.

Madison told us that she was feeling like she was "dying by inches," but because she was so good at hiding what was going on with her, few people knew she was in constant pain. As she described her experience, I was amazed that she had even showed up for the workshop. The worst thing for her was that the pain she experienced was eating up her energy. This was something that nearly everyone in the workshop could understand, since most people have experienced how pain can sap their energy and compromise their lives. Madison was a person who once had all the energy in the world; she had never dreamed her life would ever be any different. Over the previous seven years, she had built a successful consulting business, mostly on her own, but now she had to turn it over to her assistants to run, and she was afraid that things would go downhill without her direction. These necessary changes were breaking her heart, but she had no other options. She'd turned most of her attention to her recovery, searching for a way to regain the energy and well-being she had always enjoyed in the past.

I asked Madison to tell me how this had come about, seeking clues to the link between her physical conditions and the loss of energy and vitality she described.

She paused and took a deep breath before going on. Two years before, while driving home in the fog, a driver in front of her swerved to miss a road hazard and lost control of his car. Madison slammed on her brakes and managed to avoid colliding with the other car, but a split second later a delivery truck slammed into her car. Though she was badly shaken, she thought she was going to be fine, but the police ordered an ambulance and she was raced to the hospital for observation. The doctor found no broken bones or signs of other injuries, so she was released that same night and told she would be okay. All she needed was a little bed rest.

Okay turned out to be anything but. She woke up the next morning with excruciating neck and back pain. Further medical examination showed she was suffering from a classic whiplash injury, so her doctor sent her to a physical therapist. For a while, she got some relief from the stiffness, but her debilitating pain continued. She dreaded the idea of going back to work. She didn't have energy for anything. She had to force herself to even get out of bed.

When further medical tests proved inconclusive, Madison began looking for other sources of help. She tried yoga, massage, and acupuncture—all of which brought some relief, but always the energy-sapping pain returned. She found a gifted Pilates instructor who was successful in reducing the pain to a greater degree, but Madison continued to feel very constricted in her movements and limited by the pain. She felt old at forty-two. After a few sessions, her Pilates teacher told her about the work I was doing, and she signed up for the workshop.

One of the class participants, the retired doctor in the class, remarked how he'd noticed that while she stood tall and seemed flexible enough, she moved like she was walking on eggshells.

I nodded in agreement. This had been my first clue that Madison was in pain and fearful of moving. Meanwhile, her personable ways successfully masked her suffering from most people around her.

When I asked how long she'd been experiencing this pain and restriction, she looked at me with an agonized expression and answered that it felt like "ten grueling lifetimes!" Tears welled up in her eyes as she shared how she hoped this class would be helpful, since she felt it was her last hope.

I explained that to heal and become fully alive again she needed to find new ways to move, feel, and think, and the class would def-initely provide this. Her brain needed to create new patterns that excluded the pain and limitations that she was presently experi-encing. There was not a doubt in my mind that her brain could do that. I knew that the movements and other exercises I'd be guiding her through in the workshop would give her brain the information it needed to find new solutions.

Madison was worried. She explained that anything at all challenging was scary for her. She needed my assurance, which I was able to give her, that if any of the exercises I gave the class caused her any discomfort, she could just do them in her imagination. I explained that as a source of new information for our brains, imagination is often as effective and powerful as any movement exercises we perform with our bodies.

I start most of my workshops by having people lie on their backs on the floor and notice how the different parts of their bodies feel. Nothing could be simpler. But as they do this, I ask them to pay attention not just to their bodies, but also to what they are thinking and feeling emotionally. Then I have them do a very easy sequence of movements and have them pay close attention to what they are sensing in their back, rib cage, neck, shoulders, and even their eyes. They instantly begin feeling more flexible, moving in ways they hadn't been able to move for years. I ask them to stand and describe what they are feeling. Most say they feel taller and lighter on their feet. Many report that they are breathing fuller and easier. These changes, after only a few easy movements and some awareness instruction, produce outcomes that transform lifelong beliefs and experiences.

During the NeuroMovement work with Madison, I carefully watched as she did the exercises and was not surprised that she did fine with them. In fact, she did better than fine. She did all the movements attentively and gently, gradually becoming bolder, less tentative, less fearful, and far more at ease than I had imagined she would be. As we took a break, I noticed her talking excitedly with the woman next to her. Madison was sitting cross-legged on her mat, gesturing animatedly with her arms, even throwing back her head now and then to laugh. Her excitement was attracting everyone's attention.

I could barely contain my curiosity. As I walked over in her direction, she turned and looked up at me, her face radiating with sheer delight. She was already using her neck more freely. With great enthusiasm, she told me, "I can hardly believe it. My whole body feels so much better!"

The three days of class passed quickly, and as Madison was leaving she stopped to thank me. She asked if it would be possible to do some individual follow-up sessions with me. Part of her reason for this was that she wanted to stay in touch with me in case her pain returned. But there was more to it than that. "Anat," she said, "these days with you in the workshop have opened up something that feels very new in my life, and I want to learn more about it. Do you know what it is? It feels like my brain is doing something I don't think it's ever done before. It's a miracle."

I assured her that the miracle was more science than magic. It has much to do with liberating ourselves from ways of moving and acting that have become so routine and "natural" for us that we don't even think about them anymore.

Madison came in regularly for her private work with me over

the next month or two. When she came for her third session, she looked more youthful and energetic than I'd ever seen her. I told her how beautiful she looked—for she truly did—and that I was certain she was moving into her life in new and exciting ways. She laughed, nodding enthusiastically. She described how she felt "like my wild, expressive self again."

Thankfully, you don't have to experience an accident or injury to have this kind of outcome. Vitality can be awakened through my program in spite of pain from a serious injury, a chronic condition, overwork, stress, or what we often associate with "normal" aging. What Madison experienced is not an isolated or an unusual case, with or without a presenting complaint such as an injury, illness, or trauma. We have only to provide our brains with new information and new possibilities to experience renewed vitality. As our brains form new patterns, we experience a new sense of aliveness and energy, excitement, and enjoyment.

LET YOUR MIND THRIVE

In this book, you will discover that we can powerfully and quickly revitalize not only our bodies, but our mental and emotional capacities as well. Kirsten, a concert pianist and piano teacher, first came to me with a shoulder pain that she described as "maybe just a symptom of how burned out I'm feeling." As I questioned her further, I began to suspect that in addition to feeling burned out, Kirsten was seeking something important that she believed was missing from her life; as it turned out, I was right.

Her shoulder pain was gone after two private sessions. However, she signed up for weekly classes and began coming to all my longer seminars. One day, she asked if she could sign up for my professional training program, which would require a long-term commitment. I asked her why she wanted to do this, since she already had a very exciting and successful career in teaching and performing music.

She surprised me by explaining that she wanted to learn how to think better. Kirsten had been brought up in a family in which girls not only weren't expected to be smart, but were also taught not to speak out or aspire toward any kind of personal achievement. She had challenged those principles enough to become a successful teacher and musician, but she still struggled with the belief that she was not very intelligent. Because of that belief, she was inhibited in developing her intellectual skills. The ways she had learned to think about herself in her family of origin had become a barrier, but her work with me over the past months had begun removing that barrier. She had experienced profound changes in her ability to think and began feeling more confident in these abilities. She knew there was more, and she was eager to go even further and engage more fully in the intellectual and mental aspects of her life. Once she realized it was possible for her to feel and be intelligent, there was no stopping her.

In the weeks and months ahead, Kirsten began forming, trusting, and expressing her own unique understanding of life. As she continued with this process, she became more and more bold and authentic in her intellectual expression; her thinking became clearer and more creative. She often told me how empowered she felt and how much she loved the vibrancy and energy of her new intellectual life.

Today, she continues to perform and teach, bringing all she has learned as a NeuroMovement practitioner to every aspect of her life. You'll probably not be surprised to learn that she is particularly skillful at helping her students realize greater mental and creative capabilities, and bringing these to every area of their lives.

THE NINE ESSENTIALS FOR VITALITY

The *Nine Essentials for Vitality* form the core of NeuroMovement. Each of the Nine Essentials describes one of the brain's requirements for waking up and doing its job well—that is, creating new connections and avoiding rigidity and limitation. With the Nine Essentials, the brain resumes growing and changing at an incredibly fast rate, and it does so at any age and regardless of how or why it stalled, be it through illness or trauma like Madison experienced, by condition-ing such as Kirsten experienced in her youth, or by the sheer inertia of routines and habits that have lulled our brains into a haze. Once awakened, our brains resume growth and change in a way that is very similar to what we experienced as children.

As I mentioned in the introduction, until recently, it was believed that after we have grown to adulthood, our brains no longer grow very much, if at all. In fact, it was believed that past the late teens or early twenties there is a diminishing ability, or even no ability, to create new connections between various areas of the brain. We know that our brain cells start dying at a rapid rate as we approach middle age. But science has now shown that *neurogenesis,* that is, the production of new brain cells, not only occurs naturally, but can also be enhanced at any age. The adult brain retains impressive powers of neuroplasticity—the ability to change its structure and function in response to experience. For example, even with moderate athletic activity, or regular daily exercise, new brain cells start branching out, sprouting new neurons and establishing new connections with other groups of brain cells. In recent research by neuroscientist Al-varo Pascual-Leone, at the Harvard Medical School, it was shown that in learning new skills, both thinking and moving our bodies in new ways could alter the function as well as the structure of our gray matter.

My own observations with thousands of my students repeatedly confirm what these scientists report. Beyond that, it is clear to me that as our brains form new patterns, we experience a renewed sense of aliveness, energy, discovery, excitement, and enjoyment.

The Nine Essentials of NeuroMovement will help you tap into your brain's resources and open up a whole new world of possibilities. You can literally become more intelligent. You can learn to move your body better, with greater flexibility and ease. You can discover how to give and receive love more successfully.

And you can enjoy greater health, vitality, sensuality, flexibility, strength, and creativity throughout the full span of your life.

1. **MOVEMENT WITH ATTENTION.** Our brains are organized through movement. This includes movements we already know and do and movements we have yet to learn. The more habitual our everyday movements, the less we are able to satisfy the brain's need for growth. As we introduce new patterns of movement, combined with attention, our brains begin making thousands, millions, and even billions of new connections. These changes quickly translate into thinking that is clearer, movement that is easier, pain that is reduced or eliminated, and action that is more successful. As a result, new activities that we may not have even dreamed were possible become possible.

2. **THE LEARNING SWITCH.** Learning occurs in the brain. However, for the brain to do its job, the "learning switch" needs to be turned on. During childhood, the learning switch is turned on a lot. As we grow and take on the responsibilities of adulthood, we tend to develop habitual patterns, a set way of doing things, rigidity and resistance to change. Our learning switch turns off and learning slows way down. We can learn to turn the learning switch back on, regardless of age. When we do, everything in our lives becomes an opportunity, and miracles seem to pop up everywhere; our lives are filled with movement, new ideas, vivid memory, sensuality, and pleasure.

3. **SUBTLETY.** Your brain thrives on subtlety, on gentler, less-forceful, more-refined input. Conventional wisdom teaches that no pain, no gain is the way to improve or get what we want. What we discover with this Essential is that subtlety generates seemingly miraculous new possibilities that will change how you speak to your loved ones, how you present an idea, how you cook and taste, how you move, and how you remain vital. Subtlety will reveal to

you what turns your brain on and what makes it check out, instilling your life with new excitement, zest for life, creativity, and fun.

4. Variation. A life filled with possibility must include the miraculous. By trying out different ways of moving, thinking, feeling, and acting, you will become more resilient and healthy. By introducing variation into the way you move, you can end back pain. By introducing it into the way you think, you will discover new ideas and solutions that wouldn't otherwise have been possible. By introducing it into the way you feel, you awaken your senses and open doors to new worlds of sensuality and playfulness.

5. Slow. Slow gets the brain's attention and gives it time to distinguish and perceive small changes and form new connections. Fast, you can only do what you already know. To be aware and to create new patterns, you need to *feel*, and that requires slowing down. With slow, you will feel so much more, and with greater vibrancy and richness. You will immediately notice differences and have the opportunity to create new ways of moving, listening, communicating, smelling and tasting, and making love. In the words of Mae West, "If it's worth doing, it's worth doing slowly."

6. Enthusiasm. Enthusiasm is an amplifier by which you can turn up the volume, boosting the energy of everything you do, think, or feel. We often think of enthusiasm as caused by an external event. However, it can be generated from within, becoming an intentional action for transforming virtually anything in our lives. Enthusiasm can take the seemingly small, dull, boring, or unimportant and turn it into something new and magnificent. Learn to strengthen the muscle of your enthusiasm, letting the tiny become great, and you will reclaim your energy and passion.

7. Flexible goals. Goal setting is important for getting what we want from life. However, how we go about achieving our goals

can become a real impediment, creating resistance to change, *shutting us down, and even resulting in failure.* Loss of vitality, being stuck, or aging can often be traced to the way we approach our goals. By learning to hold goals loosely, you give your brain opportunities for discovering new ways to fulfill your fondest dreams. You will accomplish more, with less suffering, and open up to new possibilities. Vitality and health are fostered by adopting a free, flexible, playful attitude toward goals, embracing mistakes, and making room for miracles.

8. IMAGINATION AND DREAMS. Imagining and dreaming can transform your life. Dreams are like night vision, guiding you to create that which has never been, thus drawing you toward a yet to be discovered future. While your capacity for having a dream may become dull and jaded due to trauma, disappointment, or aging, this book will guide you in ways that will enable you to reclaim and revive this rich and vital resource any time you choose. Dreams are not "optional" if you are to fulfill your destiny.

9. AWARENESS. Awareness—knowing, and knowing that you know—is the opposite of automaticity and compulsion. Awareness means that you are in the here and now, living in the present. Awareness is a skill that we need to grow and evolve throughout life if we are to enjoy freedom and true choice. With awareness, we can have a brighter, more-cheerful, joyful, and alert life.

I encourage you to begin experimenting with the Essentials as you read and learn about them. You may work with them in the order they appear in the book, or select the ones that appeal to you most first, or the ones that you feel are most missing in your life. When you start working with the Nine Essentials, you will immediately begin experiencing the vitality that is unleashed with growth and change. The speed with which this happens may surprise you. New brain patterns and greater vitality can be established instantly, and with them you will begin to enjoy renewed energy and stamina, and a sense of well-being you may not have experienced since childhood.

In the chapters to come, we'll be exploring each of the Nine Essentials in greater depth. You will learn why these essentials work, and you'll find exercises and suggestions for experiencing the power of NeuroMovement for yourself. Some are body-movement exercises; some exercises are mental, emotional, and conceptual, not visible to the naked eye but nevertheless very real. But all address your brain, providing valuable information to help you form new patterns and new changes in your life. You may at first wonder how these small and frequently very subtle exercises and concepts can possibly make meaningful differences—but they do.

You will find yourself getting up in the morning with much more energy and the usual stiffness gone. Aches and pains you've been experiencing will be lessened. You will discover yourself getting along better with family members or difficult coworkers. You will find yourself much lighter on your feet when you walk, and walking will become really pleasurable. You will find your stamina and sensuality heightened. Your memory will be better. Thinking and problem solving will become easier, and you will more often experience the thrill of creativity and heightened intelligence. If you are active in a sport such as tennis, golf, running, or working out at the gym, you will notice yourself performing better and with greater ease and fewer injuries. Most important, you will experience yourself moving more and more fully into your life.

One

Movement with Attention—Wake Up to Life

Nothing happens until something moves.
—ALBERT EINSTEIN

Think of your life as constant movement—millions of small and large movements. Think even beyond the familiar movements associated with your bones and muscles. My teacher, Moshe Feldenkrais—a physicist and judo master who developed a revolutionary mind-body method to help people transcend their limitations—often told his students, "Movement is life; without movement life is unthinkable." Through movement, you make sounds, organized in your brain as language, that communicate to others ideas and emotions you are experiencing. Through movement, sometimes when you are alone, sometimes with others, you carry out all the activities associated with your job, profession, family, recreation, and creative expressions.

Through advanced brain research, we know that our simplest thoughts and feelings involve movement within and among billions of brain cells. Whether it's remembering that you need to pick up your dry cleaning on the way home, or feeling a surge of excitement because it's Friday, or being inspired by music you're hearing on the radio—all these involve movement. Even your daydreams and your dreams at night involve movement. The cumulative result of all this movement is who you are and what distinguishes you from me. What we begin to see as we delve into what movement means in our lives is that the quality of our movements is a manifestation of the quality of the workings of our brains and will ultimately determine the quality and vitality of our lives.

WHERE MOVEMENT IS ORGANIZED

What gives the continuous movement of our lives the particular form it takes? What organizes the ways you throw back the covers from your bed and swing your legs out to the floor as you begin each new day? What is it that organizes how you put the bread in the toaster as you are getting your breakfast? What organizes how you mutter a foggy "good morning" to your family members? What organizes your patience or impatience as you thread your way through stop-and-go commuter traffic, or how you enunciate your words or use certain facial expressions as you greet people at work? What is it that gives you the power to invent, form attitudes, and develop ideas? And what is it that orchestrates the emotional experiences you are having throughout the day?

The answer, of course, is your brain, those two to three pounds of gray matter embodied within your skull. Within your brain are billions of brain cells. Each and every one of those cells has the potential for making between five thousand and twenty thousand connections with other cells, all poised to receive and send information to and from all the various parts of your entire system. This is as close to an infinite number of possible brain connections as one can imagine. It is here in your brain that information gathered from your movements is organized, somehow making sense of the myriad messages received—and in a continuous feedback loop that also tells you how to conduct every movement you make.

Movement is the language of your brain, and your brain is the great organizer of that movement, managing trillions of connections associated with every single action, large or small. The manner in which all of this takes place will determine how you experience your life, whether you feel numbed and deadened or excited and energetic at the end of the day.

Imagine for a moment the wasted energy you'd expend if your brain organized your every step in a way that required twice the energy that would be required if your movements were better organized. Or imagine that in the process of doing its organizational tasks your brain surrounded your every thought and feeling with a million contradictions that required you to ponder, and perhaps worry over, every little thing. Life would indeed become exhausting. You'd feel drained all the time.

What we'll discover in this chapter is that the quality of organization that our brains provide us is directly related to the quality of the information we provide it. And one of the most important ways to improve the quality of the information we provide it is through *bringing attention to our movements.*

Most, if not all, experts in the health-related fields agree that movement, or what more often is referred to as exercise, is central to our health and continued well-being. We are encouraged to exercise both our bodies and our minds. Yet it is important to note that movement alone, done automatically, without attention, does not provide the brain with any new information. On the contrary, such movement will tend to groove already existing brain patterns more deeply. Over time, that leads to loss of strength and flexibility in both body and mind. We then think that we are losing our vitality due to age, life circumstances, or simply back luck. But not so. The moment we bring *attention* to our movement, any movement, research shows that the brain resumes growing new connections and creating new pathways and possibilities for us. And that is when we feel most vital.

Much of what I've learned about vitality and the brain's organizational capacities has come from working with young children born with neurological anomalies, and from adults who have suffered injuries or diseases that continue to cause them pain or a loss of normal function and vitality. Through the work I have done over the past thirty years, I've seen how profoundly important the quality of the organization of movement is—for our bodies, our thoughts, our emotions, and our feelings. Through movement with attention, we gain the ability to assist our brains in seeking the most successful way to manage all movement in our lives.

EXERCISE 1 THE TRANSFORMATIONAL POWER OF MOVEMENT WITH ATTENTION

With this simple, short exercise, you can experience firsthand the power of combining attention with movement to transform your performance and your whole sense of yourself. You can then do it in your yoga practice, sports, and everyday movements.

1. Sit at the edge of a chair with your feet comfortably flat on the floor and with about a foot of space between them.

2. Lift your right arm out in front of you, with your elbow straight but not stiff. Lift it to shoulder level and put it down two times. As you move, pay attention to how it feels. Put your arm down and stop.

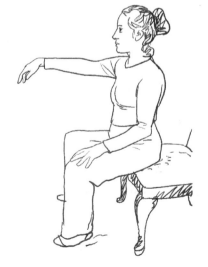

3. Now do the same movement twice with your left arm, lifting it to shoulder level, with elbow straight, paying attention to how it feels. Then lower your arm and stop.

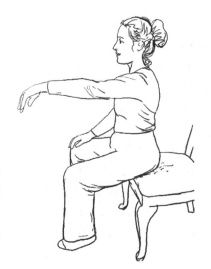

4. Select the arm of your dominant hand and do the rest of this exercise with that arm. If you are right-handed, do the exercise with that arm; if left-handed, use that arm.

5. Lift your dominant arm in front of you to shoulder level, with your elbow straight but not stiff. Keep the arm up and begin moving forward with this arm as if you were reaching for something a foot or so away. Make sure to also move forward with your upper body as you do this. Then come back to your upright sitting position. Do these reaching-out and coming-back movements two or three times.

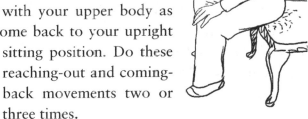

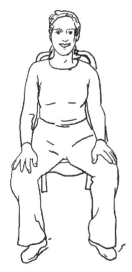

6. Stop, and come back to your neutral sitting position. Put your arm down and rest for a moment. Feel how you are sitting and how you are breathing.

7. Again, lift your dominant arm in front of you to shoulder level and reach out as you did above. Do this two or three times. But this time do something a little differently. As you reach forward and come back to your neutral sitting position, pay close attention to your lower back. Can you feel any movement there? If yes, is your lower back arching and rounding as you reach forward with your arm and come back?

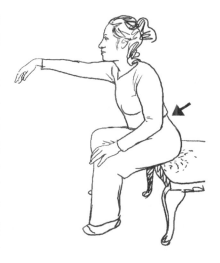

8. Stop, come back to neutral, put your arm down, and pay attention to how your shoulders feel. Does the right one feel the same as the left? If not, how do they feel different?

9. Lift your dominant arm again and continue doing the same movement as you've been doing, two or three times. But this time pay attention to your belly. For example, are you pulling in your belly when you reach forward or are you relaxing it, or perhaps pushing it out? Then pay attention to your pelvis. Do you feel movement in your pelvis as you reach with your arm and come back? If the answer is yes, are you rolling it forward when you reach out and rolling back when you come back to neutral? Stop, put your arm down, and feel how you are sitting. Do you have the impression that one arm is longer than the other? Lighter than the other? More energetic and vital?

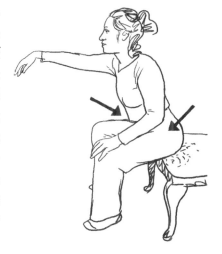

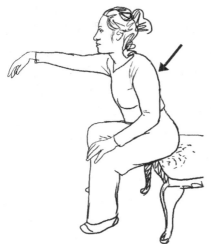

10. One more time, lift your dominant arm and do the same reaching-forward and coming back as before. This time pay attention to your ribs in your back, on the side of the arm you are lifting. Do you feel any movement in your ribs? Simply note in your mind any movement you are feeling.

11. Now, with your arm still raised and extended, reaching forward and coming back two or three times, do the following: Let your attention move, sort of like a flashlight searching in the darkness, starting with your pelvis, moving to your lower back, then to your belly, then to your chest, then to your shoulder, then to your wrist, and finally the tips of your fingers.

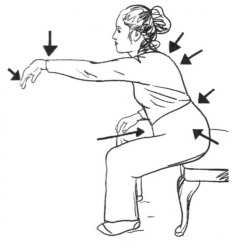

12. Stop, put your arm down, come back to neutral, and take a few seconds to notice the sensations in your body. How does your dominant arm, the arm you moved, feel? Compare it to the other arm. Do you feel any differences between the two? Feel the whole side of your body on the side you just moved—including everything from your face down to your feet. Compare these sensations to the ones on the side you didn't move and see if the two feel any different.

13. Now simply lift your dominant arm in front of you and put it down a few times. Does it feel any different than it did at the beginning of this exercise? It may feel lighter, longer, maybe larger, and perhaps you can lift it higher, with greater ease. You might feel a sense of having more energy in that arm. Now lift your other arm just one time and note whether it feels any different than your dominant arm. Does it feel heavier or clumsier? Does it seem to have less vitality?

You lift your arms many times a day, even as you are walking around and doing your usual activities. However, these arm movements do not bring about any noticeable change. In this exercise, however, which you took five minutes or so to do, you most likely are already feeling some clear changes. This is a demonstration of how the power of *movement with attention* can transform us instantly.

THE DANCE BETWEEN MOVEMENT, ORGANIZATION, AND VITALITY

Have you ever noticed that young children move nonstop when they are awake? What is all that movement about? Movement coupled with attention to the sensations, feelings, and outcomes that result serves as a rich source of new information to the brain. With every movement the child makes, new connections are taking place within their brains, forming the seemingly infinite patterns that they will use to express their lives—how they will speak, stand, run, and write, what they will think and believe and feel. Through their brains' capacities for taking in new information and organizing complex patterns, children develop their own unique capacities and ways of perceiving the world.

The relationship between movement, growth, and vitality is never so purely demonstrated as in our childhood years, when so much movement, brain activity, and formation of patterns within the brain takes place. In those first years of our lives, when we are developing so many skills and abilities, we not only move a lot, but also feel our movements vividly. This time of our lives epitomizes everything we associate with vitality—full of energy, highly flexible in body and mind, experiencing each moment as new. We are curious, optimistic, joyful, creative, inventive, and unstoppable.

At the heart of it all is movement with attention—not just movement of our muscles and bones, but also the movement that is our thinking, feeling, and emotions. By moving with attention, you will be able to resume that process of intense growth, invention, and change that we observe in children.

Every day, through the people I work with in Neuro-Movement, I see the connection between movement and vitality. By paying attention to their movements—arms, legs, torsos, eyes, how they breathe and think and feel—weariness turns to vibrancy, curiosity, and interest; rigid shoulders are suddenly freed; and locked-up emotions are liberated.

Some years ago, I worked with a woman by the name of Miriam. She was in her mid-fifties and had gone through an extremely difficult divorce a couple years before. The divorce rekindled profound pain and trauma from an extremely difficult childhood, compounding the grief and pain she was experiencing. A single mother, she found a job as an office manager and was able to create a stable financial base for her child and herself. However, she was profoundly unhappy. Hurt and disillusioned by all that life had dished out to her, she gave up on ever having another relationship, and, being depressed and shut down, she confined her life to a very limited and predictable social life, belief system, and routine.

As shut down as she appeared to be, she nevertheless attended one of my classes. She seemed to be doing okay with the movement exercises of the class and was very attentive throughout. After the class, she came to me with a big smile on her face. She explained that she wanted to thank me because she was feeling an important change in her life already.

Miriam explained that she did not understand exactly what had occurred, but as the class was progressing, she began feeling more flexible and comfortable in her body. But that was not all. "Something shifted inside me," she said. She felt as if a big weight had been lifted from her shoulders. For the first time in years, she actually felt hopeful and that her life could be different. After attending a few more classes, Miriam continued to experience changes. She moved more easily, took up swimming, and began socializing more. She was so enthusiastic about what she'd experienced that she asked me to teach in her town, which was about an hour and a half from where I lived. She was eager to have her friends experience what she was experiencing. She assured me that she knew people who would attend and would benefit greatly from taking classes with me. Because of time limitations, I had to decline, but Miriam kept asking, and one day I had an idea. I suggested that she take a training program so that she would be able to teach classes to her friends. She took me up on my offer and signed up for my next training seminar.

What followed as a result of her participating in the training was most amazing for me to watch. When she walked, she walked taller, no longer scrunched up and slightly stoop-shouldered. She walked with strong, flowing movements that exuded increased confidence. Much more than her body had begun to change; her depression and bitterness had dissolved. As she opened up emotionally, her popularity grew and she developed close friendships in the class. Her quick laughter brought a sense of levity to those around her. Her feelings, she explained, were now much more about joy and gratitude for what she did have—a beautiful daughter, health, relative security about her financial situation, and all the richness that was evolving in her life. No longer was she limited by her painful past.

Every day in the NeuroMovement workshop, she would pay close attention and observe her own movements—her thoughts and emotions as well as her body movements—and share with us the spontaneous transformations she was experiencing. The changes in her thinking, ideas, and belief system were so intense for her that for the first two weeks of the training she could hardly sleep. Time and again she exclaimed how she was feeling a freedom within herself that she had never felt before. After completing her training, she announced to her friends that she was opening her first class. A good number of people signed up.

Because of her personal experience in the training workshop she'd taken, Miriam made sure that all her students paid close attention to each movement they were doing. However, she made sure they were paying attention to more than just the movement of their bodies. Through sharing stories of her own transformation, she guided them to pay attention to what was going on in their minds, particularly to changes occurring in their emotions, their thinking, and their belief systems.

Miriam loved what she was doing, and her greatest thrill was seeing her students waking up to their lives. Her students' enthusiasm encouraged her to put more and more time into her teaching. Soon she was doing it full-time. After fifty-plus years, her life had become her own.

EXERCISE 2   GET SMART—MOVE AS YOU THINK

Since ancient times, people have associated movement with concentrated mental activity. Jews rock back and forth as they study the Torah. Socrates walked with his students as they debated complex ideas. In recent years, scientists have been able to show that movement greatly enhances the brain's ability to organize and create new connections and patterns.

As you are reading this book, sit very still, do not move, and read a few paragraphs. Then, as you continue reading, begin to gently rock back and forth or side to side. From time to time, for a few seconds, pay attention to your movements, feel the sensations in your body as you move. Does your movement with attention make it easier for you to take in what you are reading? Over the next few days, bring some movement with attention into whatever you do that requires thinking. For example, when you are trying to find a solution to a problem at work, composing a letter that is not coming out quite right, or looking for a way to ask a family member, or your boss, for a favor, at some point get up and take a walk. If walking is not an option, go where you have some privacy and do some dance steps for a few minutes. Infuse your movement with attention. Feel the sensation at the bottom of your feet, in your chest as you are breathing, and continue looking for solutions. Notice if during or after these movements with attention your thinking flows better, gets clearer, or is more creative, and whether new ideas and solutions begin to surface.

WHAT KIND OF MOVEMENT GOVERNS YOUR LIFE?

You may be thinking, "Okay, I move. There is plenty of movement in my life. I get up in the morning, do all the normal things that people do during the day. I even exercise regularly at the gym. And yet I still feel sluggish. True, I feel better for a while after working out but it doesn't last, and I don't have the vitality I once had, and certainly don't have the vitality I'd like to have today. How come?"

The first part of the answer is that life is always about movement. We all move, and do so constantly. If we didn't, we'd be dead. But is all movement alike? Clearly, it is not. There are two primary forms of movement in our lives: (1) automatic movement, and (2) movement with attention. In a very real way, vitality is a choice between these two life paths—*automatic movement* or *movement with attention*. There are many routines in our lives—from how we get up each morning to how we perform our responsibilities at work to how we swing a golf club or perform other athletic activities. These routines can be done automatically or with attention. Movement alone does not trigger vitality; movement with attention does.

First, let's look at routine or habitual movement that is done automatically. You can be involved in a very active form of exercise and movement, such as walking on a treadmill at the gym, or pumping iron, or spinning the pedals on a stationary bike for hours every week. You most likely will feel better afterward, at least for a period of time, thanks to the production of *endorphins* in your brain and to an increase in the activity both of your muscles and brain, but you may still notice little or no increase in vitality. You may feel slightly more flexible, but not significantly so, and you may even experience stiffness. Your thinking is pretty much the same; nothing new here. You are not more creative. Your relationships stay the same. Aches and pains persist, and so do your everyday thought patterns.

These activities, while stimulating the production of *feel-good* hormones such as endorphins, and providing cardiovascular and musculoskeletal benefits, are not making a sufficient difference by way of producing the kinds of connections in your brain that lead to new possibilities in your life. You can be exercising like mad—but be doing what you are doing in a way that your brain barely notices. What is missing is attention, that is, paying attention to your movements, how your body feels, any feelings of comfort or discomfort as well as pleasure that you are experiencing. Pay attention to how fast or slow you are moving, how you are breathing as you move, what you are thinking or feeling.

In a recent Vitality and Sensuality workshop, I became aware of David, a handsome man in his early thirties with a well-developed physique. He not only exercised regularly, he was also a professional fitness trainer. When I began leading the group through some simple movements, David became increasingly annoyed. He raced through every movement easily and automatically, as if to say, "These exercises are so simple they're a waste of my time."

As the group got familiar with the movements, I instructed them to pay very close attention to their movements as they were doing them. "Don't let yourself be seduced by their simplicity," I told them. I watched David's expression slowly change as his movements slowed down and he brought more attention to what he was doing. I was delighted to see that the more attention he brought to his movements, the more animated and interested he became. Then, as I finished the last day's session, he trotted up to me with a curious but spirited look in his eyes. He wanted to have a private session with me.

The following week, when he showed up at the center for his first session, I sat him down and asked what he would like from the session. He seemed shy, almost embarrassed, as he began telling me what had happened for him in the workshop. He told me that for first time in his life he felt really good about himself. He hardly knew how to talk about it except to say that he had noticed how, when he paid attention to his movements in the workshop, he began to get intrigued. There were so many feelings he'd never experienced before. He enjoyed what he was feeling. He found real pleasure in the movements themselves. Before this, he had only focused on how movements, such as working out at the gym, led to having bigger muscles and a stronger body. Now, not only were his workouts more pleasurable, he was also able to do them better than before and get better results. Paying attention to the experience of moving in the here and now, focusing his attention only on the present, was something new for him.

He'd gone home feeling energetic and that everything he did was so much easier and more enjoyable than ever before. That evening, he'd been able to connect with his girlfriend in a new way. He found spending time with her, just sharing the experiences of their day, more interesting, even more exciting, than before. Life definitely had a brighter glow for him.

The next day, he was able to do his usual fitness regime much better and more easily. He felt a breakthrough in at least one area in which he'd been limited before. He understood that it had something to do with the attention he brought to whatever he was doing, but he didn't understand why this was having such a dramatic effect on other areas of his life. He wanted to continue the process, whatever it was.

David would take one lesson, disappear for two or three weeks, and then return for another lesson. He learned to pay attention so closely that he was able to benefit from the outcome of one lesson, bring it into his daily life and his work with others, and put it into practice for a long time before he felt a need for more input from me. The central thing he was getting was how to bring his full attention to his life—to every aspect of his life, as it turned out.

For years, David explained, he had been operating on automatic pilot. He'd gotten into fitness training and the martial arts soon after high school, and these practices had become the center of his life. He developed a careful regimen that varied little from day to day. He found comfort and security in developing regular routines around these disciplines, routines by which he lived his whole life. The only trouble, he confessed, was that his life had become dull to him, and apparently to other people who were important to him, noticeably his girlfriend. He couldn't shake off his lifelong feelings of being emotionally stunted, and his movements, as nice as they looked to others, were hard for him to do. He was also experiencing aches and pains he'd never had before. All of that had now changed for him. He'd even overheard his girlfriend telling one of her friends that it was like living with a brand-new person, one who was alive and vibrant, more open and affectionate than he'd ever been. She told her friend she was falling in love all over again.

While David was unusual in his determination to change, his experience overall is not that remarkable. When we operate on automatic pilot for too long, falling into routines and habits in the ways we move, think, and even feel, we not only feel less vital, we also begin to develop real aches and pains, stuck thinking, and a certain flatness, or dullness, in our emotional and sensual lives. And, of course, we know that routines such as *repetitive exercise* can become a major source of job-related and athletic injuries.

When prolonged over many years, routine living becomes a rut. To the people around us—as well as to ourselves—we become predictable and lackluster. By sheer inertia, we may find ourselves resisting any suggestions that might change how we think, feel, or do things. We resist even our own desires to pull ourselves out of our rut. We all tend to do this, in either small or large ways. It's just human. But it does lead to the inertia in which we can lose ourselves in repetition and sameness. Living too much out of habit and routine blinds us to new experiences, which our brains crave and which, in truth, can be found in every moment of our lives. Blinded by habit and routine, we are often left with the impression that there is nothing new, nothing to get excited about, nothing to say, do, or feel that hasn't been said, done, or felt a million times before. In short, we cease to find anything that would trigger new growth and new connections in our brains.

We all know how, after years of maintaining certain routines, movements that are done over and over again in the same way become restricted, no longer evolving. This inevitably leads to joint pain and muscular soreness. Much of the time in my work with adults, people come to me because they are in pain or because they cannot comfortably do things they once did easily and for pleasure. This can include everything from carpal tunnel syndrome, for people who spend long hours keyboarding or doing other repetitive movements with their hands and arms, to certain arthritic conditions and to back, shoulder, and neck pain. Along with these conditions, they may have a generalized feeling that it is difficult to initiate movement, and there is no longer pleasure in moving. Not surprisingly, pain and physical discomfort affect our emotional and intellectual lives, limiting our responsiveness to the world around us. All such restrictions result in a loss of vitality.

The good news is that we do not need to be trapped by routine and its painful or otherwise limiting side effects. When we bring our attention to our movements—body, mind, and emotions—our brains are able to use the new information that movement with attention provides to transform the unwanted condition. With attention, better-organized movements are introduced and discomfort disappears and we experience well-being and vitality.

EXERCISE 3   THE MOVEMENT OF YOUR EMOTIONS

You are probably familiar with the popular expression "I was moved" when commenting on emotional experiences. What's expressed in this common saying is our innate awareness of emotion as movement. (Think "E-motion," that is, "energy in motion.") Just as bringing attention to the movement of our bodies brings about change and increased vitality, so too bringing attention to our emotions can bring about greater freedom, increasing our energy and our sense of well-being where our emotional life is concerned. To appreciate this, choose a situation in your life in which you experience strong emotions. For example, maybe there's a scene in a favorite movie that has always moved you in a certain way, or a TV program whose stories or characters move you, or certain political topics that get you riled up. Or perhaps you experience strong emotions associated with your communication with your child, another family member, or a coworker. Next time you are in one of these situations, pay close attention to your emotions as you experience them and observe how they begin to change. For example, you might feel angry at someone in your life, but then, as you pay close attention, your feelings slowly transform into compassion, even love. As you get more skillful at paying attention to the movement of your emotions, you will notice how *good* feelings tend to get richer and fuller, spreading throughout your whole being. You will also notice how *bad* feelings tend to tone down, with new emotions emerging. To bring vitality into your emotional life, simply pay attention, from time to time throughout the day, to the movements of your emotions.

THE POWER OF ATTENTION

In recent years, there has been an explosion of research showing how brain activity radically changes when we bring attention to even a routine movement. This phenomenon has been known and practiced in many spiritual traditions for centuries. In his book *The Power of Now,* on Buddhist practices in modern life, Eckhart Tolle writes that the more consciousness, or attention, we direct toward our movements, the higher the "vibrational frequency becomes, much like a light that grows brighter as you turn up the dimmer switch and so increase the flow of electricity."

What Tolle states intuitively can now be stated scientifically as well. Each time we combine attention with movement, millions and millions of brain cells are activated. Imagine for a moment that you have the capacity to look inside your head and see the trillions of brain cells, each one like a tiny lightbulb that becomes brighter when active. At rest, all the cells emit a nice, faint glow, with those controlling your muscles and other organs of your body glowing a little bit brighter than the rest. Now you begin moving, perhaps just your right arm. Suddenly, a cluster of cells begins glowing brighter and brighter. When you stop moving, the lights dim back down.

Now you move your arm as before. Approximately the same cluster of brain cells lights up. Then you add a new element: *attention.* No longer running on automatic pilot, you are now aware and awake, experiencing your movements with your five senses and your mind. You turn this attention to how it feels to move your arm, as well as how fast, slow, or far you extend it. With attention, the brain's organizational functions are spurred into action. Now you see brand-new clusters of cells lighting up, in many different areas of your brain. You might even imagine, at this point, something like an artfully choreographed fireworks display, as clusters of brain cells begin communicating with one another, exchanging information and reorganizing the patterns of the clusters so that they will signal more refined movements of your arm.

As improbable as it might seem, this metaphorical play of energy and lights offers a pretty accurate mental image of what happens in our brains as we move and bring attention to our movements. The more we combine attention with movement, the greater the number of brain cells that *light up,* joining to form new patterns to create new possibilities for our lives, be it a new action, a new idea, a different feeling or emotion, or new knowledge.

As we've seen in David's story, when a person continues to follow the path of movement with attention, every area of his life begins to change. Life becomes more interesting and exciting again. He finds greater pleasure in physical activities; his sensuality is awakened; his emotional life becomes more vibrant; and even his belief systems open up to new ideas. The one overriding benefit, however, is increased vitality, which is apparent to those around him the moment he walks into a room. How could one not notice someone with billions of brain cells lit up!

EXERCISE 4   ATTENTIVE HAND

Next time you touch your partner or begin caressing her or him, pay close attention to the movement of your own hand. Notice how this movement feels across your palm and fingers as your hand moves over the contours of your partner's body. Take in the sensations of your joined energy as your hand moves. Notice the changing qualities of your touch as your sensations begin to transform for you and your partner; that is, be aware of how, as both of your sensations are awakened, you become more attentive to each other and your experience of each other deepens in the moment.

THE SEDUCTIVENESS OF ROUTINE
AND HABIT

While our brains are truly miraculous in their ability to process information, and invent and organize complex movement, they are also excellent at creating set "templates" or "programs" that allow us to do routine activities very well. In fact, our brains are so good at creating programs and templates that we can go through virtually any of our everyday activities on automatic pilot and lose all awareness of where we are or what we are doing. I've certainly had this experience while working out at the gym. After a difficult day, I admit, it can be a relief to just go on automatic pilot and tune out the world in this way. Many of my students have explained that they plug themselves into their iPods so they can listen to music or recorded books, or even watch TV, as they are working out at their local gym or health club. No doubt about it, tuning out helps to pass the time as we give our bodies the exercise they need to stay fit. The main function of our brains at this time is to provide the set patterns—templates and programs—to follow existing routines.

These habits and routines have enormous value. We couldn't live without them. They provide us with ways to do things reliably, efficiently, and safely. Think of how impossible life would become if we had to learn anew every activity in our lives, from getting out of bed in the morning to walking down the street!

We have spent many years learning all the things that we do today so we can do them effectively and without too much conscious thought. We used repetition in a conscious and deliberate way to master a new skill in our profession, or in an athletic activity, or in any of a million other activities. But the one ingredient we bring to repetition as we learn to master a new skill is our attention—attention to how we are constructing each sentence if you're a writer, or how you are swinging the racquet if you're playing tennis, or how you are modulating your voice if you're a singer.

Once we've developed our skills sufficiently, we may maintain a routine activity with that skill. However, unless we also remind ourselves, again and again, to bring our attention to the movements—intellectual, emotional, and physical—that are involved in that activity, we begin stagnating. We will bring less and less energy and awareness to what we are doing. Our brain's organizational activities will then diminish and our vitality will erode, giving way to weariness and boredom. We become less and less aware of the world around us, content just to stick with our routines, going down pretty much the same track day after day, producing exactly the opposite of what we are seeking—vitality.

We easily slip into robotic periods of activity in daily routines, particularly with those household tasks and everyday jobs that we perform as a matter of course. Whether at home, at work, or at play, our set ways of doing things can become so routine that one day begins to feel pretty much like another. With the same old movements, and no attention brought to those movements, no new information is fed to our brains; thus, few new patterns are created. The patterns that once organized our movements so well begin to degrade. As one student put it, *after a while it's like nobody's home.*

Some people call this state of being "burnout time." We've all been there at one time in our lives. One of the first things we then hear from friends, and even our therapists and doctors, is "A change of scene will do you wonders." We consider taking a trip to Europe, or leaving for a weekend at some romantic getaway. Or maybe we should change jobs or change friends or move to a new town where nobody knows us. Any of these changes can be fun and exciting, but too often we change our surroundings and yet bring along the same old routines and habitual ways of acting and responding that got us into a rut in the first place. We need to constantly remind ourselves that vitality comes about by bringing attention to our movements.

BREAK OUT OF ROUTINE

We need to notice, and focus our attention, on *what* we are doing, *how* we are moving our bodies, *how* we are thinking, and *what* we are feeling. The moment we bring attention to any movement, brain activity increases and new connections are made and strengthened, specifically the brain's organizational abilities.

Our brains crave new information—and a lot of it. When routine becomes the predominant way of being in our lives, and our brains don't get their needs met, even our moods change; stress increases, and soon we feel drained at the end of the day. The longer we live our routine automatically, the more resistant we become to any change in the routine. We all know the frustration we experience when our most habitual routines are interrupted. When the unexpected intrudes—be it anything from finding there's no coffee in the morning to being told we're being downsized at our job—we can become quite upset. We don't know where to turn. We may feel lost, frightened, or even depressed.

The less we are bound to routine, the broader our experience tends to be, and when our routines are interrupted, or life challenges intrude, we have more resources to draw from. We are confident that beyond our routines are infinite possibilities just waiting to be discovered.

The good news is that you can bring this kind of attention into your life this very moment and once again see the world anew, with all kinds of new possibilities. You needn't go anywhere, buy anything, rearrange your furniture, change your hairstyle, or seek new friends. The secret is right there—in your head.

MOVE INTO LIFE

I recently heard a ninety-seven-year-old woman interviewed on the radio. With a strong, resonant, highly expressive voice, she was

telling about a book she was writing and which she looked forward to having published next year. She also spoke of the many
lectures she had given over the past few years, and how she had integrated into her book what she had learned from other women
during Q & A sessions after her talks. In her work, she was exploring what it meant to live a full and vital life. Obviously, she
was walking her talk. Here was a woman of advanced years who
was a living example of what it meant to have an active, creative,
energetic, and personally gratifying life.

She was scheduled, in two months, to fly to China, where she
would be delivering a lecture and speaking with other women at
an international women's conference. She appeared to be a person
whose mind was alive with new ideas, new observations about
life, and new insights about herself. At ninety-seven, she was still
fully engaged in life, excited, articulate, and fun. She spoke of how
much she had learned from other women in her lectures and inter-
views for the book, and how every day was filled with new ideas.

When asked what she thought the secret of her vitality and
longevity might be, she said she could not answer that for certain.
She talked a little about watching her diet, but only insofar as she
ate fresh, good-quality food, and occasionally a cookie or two.
Over the years, she had learned techniques for managing stress, including meditation, cognitive therapy, and movement to manage
stress. "Movement" was key—movement of her body, her mind,
and her ideas, movement with attention, leaving room for change
and growth in the way she thought and felt. She realized that just
as she could have a stuck pattern in her body, she could also have
a stuck thought or emotion that no longer moved, was always the
same. She actively sought new ideas through reading books, seeing
movies, listening to music, going to museums, and listening to
people who challenged her own beliefs and feelings, and—most
important—she made sure she paid attention to her own thoughts
and emotions. Listening with attention to music that was new to
her introduced new feelings to her brain. Listening with attention
to new ideas and beliefs moved her brain to create new ideas of

her own. The result was greater flexibility in her mental and emotional capacities—greater ability to be *present, in the now,* constantly creating new possibilities that kept life open and vital.

Louis Armstrong, the great jazzman, used to sing a blues song that went "It ain't what you do, it's the way how you do it, that's what gets results!" The concept he expressed here reminds us that if we organize the notes of a piece of music one way, we get chaos and want to cover our ears; organize the same notes another way and we get an exquisite, moving, wildly exciting experience that makes us happy to be alive. Remember, all life is movement; thus, we can think of our brains as the great composers of the notes, the daily actions, the thoughts, and the feelings that comprise our lives.

Our brains are in charge of all the movement in our lives. How those movements are organized, poorly organized, or disorganized, as the case may be, will have an enormous impact on our lives. When the organization is working well, we feel fully alive, free of pain, creative, moving in ways that are fluid and easy. Most of the complaints associated with loss of vitality—stiffness, pain, lack of energy, mental lethargy, loss of interest, or diminished excitement about our lives—can be traced to *poor organization* in the movements in our brains.

All of us develop ways of thinking, feeling, and acting that include some level of disorganization. This may come about because we grew up in a difficult environment, or because we suffered physical trauma, or because of a serious illness, or because we have experienced the stresses of life, or simply because we didn't know there was a way for us to do it better. Whatever the circumstance, movement with attention will change how our brains put it all together. Our human destiny, if we're to be vital and alive and healthy, is to keep creating those opportunities for change and growth by choosing, over and over again, to bring movement and attention to all that we do.

Exercise 5   Movement with Attention

What's Your Vitality Quotient?

On a scale of 1 to 5, rate yourself on each of the following statements, with 5 being always, 3 being occasionally, 1 being never.

1. I jump at opportunities to move, whether it's taking the dog for a walk or taking the stairs instead of the elevator.

2. I have a regular exercise program and participate in it several days a week.

3. From time to time during the day, I pay attention to how I am performing daily actions, whether it's pouring my coffee into a mug or sitting in my favorite chair.

4. I take mini breaks throughout the day to check in with myself and bring my attention to any discomfort I might be feeling in my body.

5. When I feel anger, irritation, or impatience with another person, I pay close attention to the emergence and movement of these feelings.

6. Whenever I encounter mentally challenging situations, I take movement breaks to improve my thinking.

7. Throughout the week, I pay attention to any habits or routines I've established and look for new ways of doing them.

Score Yourself
24–35 points = high
15–23 points = medium
1–14 points = low

Go through the seven statements above and choose the ones on which you scored the lowest. Take some time to think about ways to improve your scores in those areas. The statements themselves will guide you.

Two

The Learning Switch—
Bring in the New

Live as if you were to die tomorrow. Learn as if you were going to live forever.

—Mahatma Gandhi

Healthy young children at play are the very essence of vitality. We see in their faces, their wide-eyed wonder, their seemingly boundless energy, and their sheer joy and excitement with each moment something that we adults have either lost or fear we might lose. Through working with thousands of people, from all age groups, over thirty years, I've found that the child's vitality is the product of a very specific state of being. Moreover, I have helped my many clients initiate this state of being through a process I call *turning on the learning switch.* One thing is very clear—the boundless vitality of children is not just a nostalgic notion but is a particular way of being in the world, one that we can all bring into our lives on a consistent and reliable basis.

By now it should be clear to you that the loss of vitality is not something that happens only because of the passage of time. Yet many people experience some loss of vitality beginning quite early in life, even as early as their teens. What is it that so often reduces our vitality as we grow up, take on new responsibilities, and settle into a routine? This loss is related to the fact that along the way we learn the disciplines of everything from toilet training to getting a college education. We develop means for dealing with emotional and physical demands. As time goes by, we learn a trade or we go off to college to learn a profession. Mixed together with all these things are the beliefs we adopt around politics, religion, life values, and simply getting along with other people. All of this is fine and well. But there's a hurdle that gets created along the way, one that we need to soar over if we are to enjoy lives lavished with vitality. Once again, we find the answers by looking at how our brains work.

The human brain is geared for efficiency, for getting its work done as simply, directly, reliably, and quickly as possible. When we are introduced to any new activity—crawling or walking, for a child, or learning a new language or a new dance step for an adult, for example—new synapses are created at a rapid rate and in large numbers, and we become vibrant. Yet, over a period of time, as we refine that activity, our brains start choosing the most efficient pathways for doing it and lets go of millions of extra synapses that are not required for performing that activity efficiently through a process that brain researchers call "pruning."

In 1949, a researcher by the name of Donald Hebb proposed that it is through gaining experience in an activity that this pruning occurs. His theory can be stated as "cells that fire together, wire together"; that is, cells that constantly work together will, over time, join in persistent patterns. This phenomenon, in which the plasticity of the brain coupled with repeated experience actually reduces the number of connections in the brain, has been named *Hebbian plasticity*. Some researchers refer to these patterns as "grooves" guiding the flow of information. While forming these efficient patterns in everything in our lives—from learning to walk, run, read, write, do math, and relate to others all the way up to developing efficiency in jobs, professions, and recreational activities—is not just normal but necessary, there's another side to all this that we can't ignore. As these grooves form, they tend to protect their own integrity by rejecting neurons that might alter those patterns. Essentially, the grooves resist new learning.

Our brains create order out of what otherwise would seem like utter chaos. As they take in stimuli and organize them into useful patterns—that is, information—we develop an inner vision, or model, of what our world is about. When these patterns are successful enough, our brain then imposes that model, or vision, on the external environment and on our experience. The brain takes in stimulation from the world around us and within us, and organizes it according to knowledge it already has. Everything we have learned, and that we hold in our brains, comes into play to "make sense of" the world. While it may seem that a ball is really round or a box really square, that one thing is *good* and another is *bad,* that certain situations are threatening and others safe, it is our brain that has learned to interpret them as such. What we hold in our brains may even determine the possibilities we see or fail to see for our lives.

The story is often told that when Magellan and his crew landed in the Pacific islands, the natives asked how they had gotten there. When the sailors pointed to their large ships on the horizon, the natives could not see them. Though there was nothing wrong with the natives' eyesight, the large ships were invisible to them. Their brains simply lacked the information to make sense of what they saw—or didn't see—out there. They lacked the brain patterns the Europeans obviously had to impose the meaning of "ship" on the visual stimuli they saw out there bobbing around on the ocean waves.

As often as not, this capacity of our brains to impose order and meaning on the world works well for us. We see an obstacle in the road in front of us. Our brains immediately respond: "Danger, slow down!" Instantly, we start drawing upon knowledge already stored in our brains; we slow down, and from the information organized in our brains we safely dodge the obstacle and go safely on our way. When we see a glass of water, we reach for it in a way that is already known to us, recognizing what's inside the glass and the purpose of its contents. When our child suddenly cries, we know to stop what we are doing and attend to him or her.

Our brains also impose themselves on human relationships, often with less than perfect results. How many times have you found yourself interpreting another person's behavior in a way that turned out to be wrong? For example, when she was growing up and anyone in her family got sick, Harriet's family showered the sick person with close and constant attention. Jed's family took care of the sick person by giving them as much peace and quiet as possible. Their way of caring was to stay in the background most of the time while being attentive to anything he or she asked for. So the first time Harriet got sick after they married, Jed did what he'd learned to do—leave her alone and wait for her to ask him for things. She was crushed, believing Jed didn't love her anymore. This is a clear example of how our brains impose preexisting patterns on the world, and we each do it all the time.

When we only rely on what we already know—or what we believe we know—we create the same experiences for ourselves over and over again, no matter what comes our way. We all need to create some degree of predictability or we'd never be able to accomplish anything; however, if we become too rigid in our efforts to create this predictability, we are sure to inhibit our vitality. You have probably had the experience of being with somebody in a new place who is constantly saying, "Oh, this is just like at home," or "Doesn't this music remind you of that TV program we saw yesterday?" This tendency to equate every new experience to something we already know deadens our vitality in everything from greeting our partners in the morning to making love with them at night.

It may be true that you are in a place that reminds you of home. And it might be true that the music is like the music you heard on the TV program. And maybe your morning greetings and lovemaking are predictable morning and night. But that needn't be so. These are simple examples of imposing on the moment at hand that which you have experienced and learned in the past. Over time, this easily becomes a habit, and the more habitual it becomes, the less you will tend to create something new. Unless we give our brains the opportunity to perceive new stimuli and create new information, pretty soon every moment of our lives will start looking like every previous one. Our lives will soon be wrung dry of any sense of vitality. The state of mind at work in a situation like this is the direct opposite of the state of mind we observe in the healthy child and the vital adult for whom each moment brings something new.

One of the first signs that our brains are rigidly using the same, existing patterns, imposing the old on the new, over and over again, is boredom. When we stop rigidly imposing what we already know on the world, something very different begins to happen. Just as with healthy children, our brains begin working with the stimulation entering the brain to create new information and new possibilities. This is a pivotal point, and it is here that we discover an important secret that opens doors to achieving lifelong vitality—*turning on the learning switch*, one of our Nine Essentials.

Exercise 1   Been There, Done That

Much of the time, we try to make sense of our life experience by comparing the present with the past. Our brains are made this way, and interpreting the present based on the past serves us well much of the time. For example, if you step off the curb and see a speeding truck bearing down on you, you instantly interpret this as dangerous and run for safety. While interpreting the present through the lens of past experience is normal and healthy, trying to fit our current experience into the mold we are familiar with shuts off our learning switch. If the present only echoes the past, our brains go on automatic, as if asleep; we stop creating anything new, life becomes humdrum, and we ourselves grow quite boring.

The tendency to interpret the present from the past shows up in subtle ways. How often have you thought, or heard yourself say of a new experience, "This is like . . .," or "This reminds me of . . .," or "Doesn't she look just like . . .," or "All men (or women) are alike," or "Here we go again!" This might occur while visiting a new place, having dinner with friends, trying to resolve an issue with your boss or coworker, or even while making love with your partner. When you think or speak in these ways, you make the present be just like the past. Your actions will tend to be habitual and predictable. You shut down your learning switch and loose the burst of energy that comes with discovery, creativity, and invention.

When you have the experience of sameness, try to identify anything that is different for you. This might be a small detail, such as how your body feels or how you are moving. Perhaps you will notice an expression on your lover's face that you have never noticed before, or a reaction to your touch that you haven't perceived before that will lead you to be more creative in your lovemaking. Or maybe at work you'll hear something new in your boss's communication that will motivate you to work with that person in a whole new way. You will be amazed how the discovery of that one different thing will frequently lead you to experience the present situation as unique. You bring yourself into the present, your brain wakes up and starts creating new patterns, and you become more vital.

THE SWITCH

I will never forget the first time I became aware of the learning switch. It was more than thirty years ago, and I was working with a new client. Katie was a professional caterer. Her business partner, who had attended one of my classes, had strongly encouraged Katie to see me. Katie had been finding it harder and harder to do her job. Even though she had no critical complaint, she fatigued faster, found it difficult to be on her feet for many hours, and at the end of her work day felt achy and lacked interest in doing anything. She was too tired and complained that her body felt leaden.

When Katie walked into my office for the first time, I observed that she moved in a somewhat rigid manner. As I looked into her eyes, and watched her face, I had the impression of a thin veil between the two of us that was somehow preventing her from connecting with me in any significant way. You have probably had that experience when talking with a friend and you suddenly realized they were barely participating in the conversation. You might have even found yourself wanting to say, "Hello? Is anybody home in there?" That is how it was with Katie. As she explained why she came to see me, she was friendly and polite, but I noted that her responses to my questions were flat, lacking vibrancy. She was there and not there. I was connecting with her, but she was not connecting with me.

When I am working with individual clients like Katie, I use movement exercises like those in the book, except that I'm guiding their movements with my hands. As I first touched her body, it felt like a block. I realized that Katie had been doing her job, using her body like a reliable machine for nearly twenty years, performing many of the same tasks in the ways she had learned long ago. As I was touching her body and moving it gently, leading her through some new configurations of movement, it was as if she were melting under my hands. Her back, arms, and legs became light and increasingly flexible, moving more fluidly and harmoniously. Katie was paying close attention to what she was experiencing as I did my work. Ten or fifteen minutes into that first session, her face started to change. It became far more expressive, and there was more vitality in her responses. I was a very young teacher at the time, and I was both puzzled and intrigued by what was happening. The more I worked with her, the more she lost the dull, glazed-over look she first had in her eyes and the more I felt that we were connecting.

Several days later, as I welcomed her into my office for her second session, she actually greeted me with enthusiasm, and I noticed that her face was more animated than in our first session. My impression of there being a thin veil separating us was nearly gone. Katie told me that she already felt some changes while at work. It took longer before she felt fatigued, and her body did not ache as much at the end of the day. She even went to the movies one evening with her husband.

During this second session, I immediately noticed that she was participating in a new way. She asked lots of questions, was interested in what I was doing with her, and from time to time told me what she was feeling as I was working with her. At the end of the session, while saying good-bye, I noticed that the veil between us was completely gone. As I walked home that evening, the image of Katie's newly animated and expressive face popped into my mind. I realized at this moment that through my touch, and through Katie's movements and her close attention to those movements and her feelings, it was as if she had turned on an imaginary switch in her brain—the learning switch. I began to understand that we come to life when we turn on the learning switch.

I then thought of the biblical quote about mouths that do not speak, eyes that don't see, and ears that don't hear. With each new session, Katie was becoming more alive. Her responses told me that *her brain was eagerly turning the stimuli I presented in our sessions into new information* that led to rapid changes and improvements. Katie also turned on her learning switch at work. Her brain was at the ready to form new patterns that left her with more energy at the end of the day. Her ears were hearing, her eyes were seeing, her body was feeling, and her mind was thinking. Where once she had been stuck and expressionless, she now became responsive and expressive.

By her third and subsequent sessions, she was arriving poised to learn. Any impression of a veil separating us had vanished. What I saw instead was a nearly palpable sense of positive expectation. I remember telling a friend that it almost didn't matter what I did when Katie's learning switch was on. I could sneeze and her brain would somehow convert it into information that would be valuable for her. Once her learning switch was turned on, her vitality radically improved. Not only was she more vibrant and expressive, but she reported that she was much more innovative at her job, was sleeping better, moving more flexibly, and enjoying life more than ever before.

For the first time, it struck me that when a client's learning switch was turned off, no amount of my work with her would produce much benefit. When it was turned on, change occurred as if by some miracle, and with it came a very high level of vitality.

More and more I noticed the same phenomenon with my other students, both in private sessions and workshops. Whether they were six months old or eighty, it was always the same. As soon as the learning switch turned on, the impression of the veil dissolved. Their faces not only became lively and expressive, but their presence also shifted from a passive state into a state of anticipation, curiosity, inquiry, and discovery. They were meeting each moment as fresh and new, and they hungrily took in new stimuli and began creating new possibilities for themselves. Like turning on a switch that fills a dark room with light, turning on the learning switch fills our lives with vitality.

EXERCISE 2   BEGINNER'S MIND—TURNING ON YOUR LEARNING SWITCH

You are probably familiar with the term "beginner's mind," which has come into the popular lexicon from Buddhist teachings. It simply means voluntarily suspending anything we think we know. You might think of it as having the kind of vibrant and open mind we had as young children, always with the learning switch turned on.

Select a situation or area in your life in which you feel stuck and into which you want to bring more vitality. This might be in a relationship at home or at work, a financial situation, your exercise routine, communications with your children, an education or career change, or perhaps something as big as taking a new look at your life values and beliefs. Choose an issue that is real, in which the outcome is important to you.

Switch to beginner's mind. Take the position that the issue in which you feel stuck is new to you and you don't have any prior knowledge of it. Is this too big of a jump, since you do have some knowledge regarding this issue? How about that you agree that you don't presently know how to handle this situation as well as you'd like and that some new knowledge could be useful? What we learn from beginner's mind is that we usually get stuck because we try to solve our problems by applying the same beliefs and behaviors that created the problem in the first place.

Take a moment or two and focus your attention very lightly on whatever issue you have chosen to work on. Suspend all effort to solve anything about that issue. In fact, take the position that any knowledge you presently have about it is either incomplete or getting in the way of a resolution. Be in beginner's mind, letting it be okay to *not know*.

As you step into beginner's mind, shift your focus to something you have recently experienced but which is unrelated to your issue. It could be as mundane as a bit of conversation you've overheard in a restaurant, a scene from a movie, a song on the radio, a story a friend shared, or the grace you felt when working out at the gym. See if anything in these situations inspires new ideas regarding your issue.

With beginner's mind, solutions often come from unexpected places and circumstances. The learning switch is turned on, and the brain is free to create unexpected new connections and new solutions.

Over the next few days, continue to repeat this exercise two or three times a day, again focusing on your issue. Each time, bring in new associations that seem unrelated to that issue, creating the opportunity for the unexpected to occur.

You can bring beginner's mind not just to what you know you don't know, or where you feel stuck, but also to what you think you already know very well. In fact, bringing beginner's mind to those areas in which you are most experienced can be tremendously fruitful, vitalizing that area of expertise and your whole life with increased energy and creativity.

TURN ON THE LEARNING SWITCH

In the early stages of my career, the learning switch of my students seemed to turn on serendipitously. I did not know what turned it on or what turned it off. But I soon learned that there were things I could do to make this process intentional. What's more, it was relatively easy for people to learn how to turn on the learning switch for themselves; and when they did, their whole lives changed. They moved into life in a new way, with great enthusiasm and pleasure. With the learning switch turned on, we fill every moment with life, rather than living by habits, routines, and sameness.

When I reflect on the quality of life people experience when the learning switch is on, I recall that wonderful and popular picture of Albert Einstein, in his seventies at the time, wheeling playfully around the Princeton campus on his bicycle, a huge grin on his face as he weaves around students and various obstacles. There's a quote attributed to him during this time that I dearly love: "Life is like riding a bicycle. To keep your balance you must keep moving." To keep moving into life—and to keep the flame of vitality always burning—it is important to learn how to turn the learning switch on and keep it on.

In recent years, there has been much talk, and many books written, about the importance of lifelong learning and what author-psychiatrist Daniel G. Amen calls "Brain Workouts" in keeping our brains young and healthy through mental exercise. In his book *Making a Good Brain Great*, Dr. Amen cites more than three decades of work by neuroscientist Marian Diamond, of the University of California at Berkeley, showing how certain conditions keep our brains healthy well beyond our retirement years. Dr. Diamond has stated, "We now know that with proper stimulation and an enriched environment, the human brain can continue to develop at any age."

Learning plays an important part in Dr. Amen's prescription for keeping our brains active. He suggests taking classes about something you find new and interesting, improving skills you already know, breaking routines in your life, making love in new ways, trying a new sport, learning new cooking recipes, going to concerts to hear music that is new to you, joining a personal development group, learning new words, making a new friend, and visiting new places. In addition to Dr. Amen's work in this area, there are numerous books and workshops prescribing "brain calisthenics," including doing crossword puzzles, taking ballroom dancing, learning to play Ping-Pong, and avoiding foods and drugs that are toxic for your brain.

The success of such programs provides evidence that the human brain loves new challenges and new learning, and will continue to stay healthy as long as you feed it what it needs. All of this new thinking around keeping the brain young is indeed invaluable.

Yet, the extent to which such activities will enhance new growth in our brains will depend on how fully our learning switch is turned on as we participate in them.

Whether being exposed to new situations will increase our vitality will depend on how we approach new stimuli, be it a brain puzzle, a new job, a new relationship, a new yoga pose, or a trip to exotic lands. To make use of this fact, you need to know the three types of learning, what they have to do with vitality, and how we can apply it in our own lives.

WHAT KIND OF LEARNER ARE YOU?

Some years ago, the concept of learning styles became popular among educators. They showed how there are visual learners, who learn primarily through seeing and processing imagery; auditory learners, who learn primarily through listening; and kinesthetic learners, who learn primarily through movement, doing, and touching. None of us are purely one style of learner or another; however, if you know your preferred style, you can use it to facilitate your own learning.

I have realized in my work that we not only have these different ways of taking in and processing information—visually, auditorily, or kinesthetically—but that there are also three broad approaches to learning that affect how our brains organize information and the quality and degree to which they will grow and change. These are *academic learning, skill acquisition,* and *organic learning.*

> *First you know and then you learn.*
> —MOSHE FELDENKRAIS

Academic learning is about acquiring new information. A simple example of this would be learning the dates of historical events. With academic learning in its simplest form, we are learning something that already exists as a *known* or *accepted fact,* with the intention of continuing to hold this knowledge for the future. The academic may even function as a gatekeeper, maintaining standards so that valuable knowledge is not lost or corrupted. Recognize, of course, that as we advance in academic learning, the process may be much more than this, resulting in the creation of new knowledge and deepening our understanding of a particular subject. But for our use here, think of academic learning in its simplest form, of learning information by rote.

Skill acquisition is learning a new skill or activity. Examples of this include learning to swing a golf club, or to ski, or to play tennis, learning a new language, or learning how to operate a new software program at work. Initially, skill acquisition is very different from academic learning. We are learning to do something that we couldn't do before, so we ourselves are involved and are changing. We thus have to pay some attention to ourselves and how this new thing we're learning is affecting us. We've got to make it somewhat personal. For example, we may begin by learning the basic principles and movements of skiing. We need to learn how to execute the moves and, because we are trying them for the first time, we have to notice what our bodies are doing and overcome any trepidations we might have. We are personally involved. But we can learn a skill in such a way that it is as if we are learning something outside ourselves. Our own abilities, inclinations, handicaps, fears, or physical capacities are hardly taken into account during the learning process. If the activity is learned without consideration for the uniqueness of our own bodies, hearts, and minds, the activity can later actually reduce our vitality. For example, I have helped musicians who later in life developed musculoskeletal problems as a result of early teaching that failed to address the whole person. If we get full engagement (making certain the learning switch is turned on) in the early stages of learning a new skill, we learn faster and become more accomplished in that skill, and our brains are stimulated in ways that lead to personal transformation, with all its attendant benefits for maintaining and boosting vitality.

Organic learning is any learning that brings about personal change, and this cannot occur until the learning switch is turned on. Whenever we have participated in organic learning, we know that it has changed us in meaningful ways. We feel and act different. Something new is going on not only outside us, but also inside us. To learn organically, we need to approach each moment as unique and new. It is personal in the sense that in the process of learning, something new is revealed to us about ourselves and the world around us, involving our thoughts, our beliefs, and the way we move and feel. Our brains do something qualitatively different from what we normally do. Instead of imposing sameness on the experience, our brains switch on and create something new.

The experience of vitality associated with organic learning comes, in part, from being intimately connected with the moment. This results from bringing ourselves into the equation, expecting it to be different from anything that has gone before. You have a willingness to be vulnerable, that is, to allow yourself to be changed by new experience.

Many years ago, I worked with a famous orchestral conductor for the Boston Symphony Orchestra who not surprisingly turned out to be a most amazing organic learner. I was teaching at the Boston Symphony's Tanglewood Music Festival at the time that this maestro was giving a concert. He was referred to me because he'd been having trouble with his right shoulder, which was naturally of considerable concern to him. When he came to me, he was very curious about what I was doing. It was very new to him. I answered his questions, and as I began working with him, he quickly moved into total engagement with the process.

He reported after the session that his right arm and shoulder felt lighter and moved more fluidly and easily than ever before. He was confident he would be fine for that night's concert. That evening, I was in the back of the auditorium to listen to the music. The conductor came out, bowed to the audience, took his position before the orchestra, and tapped his baton on the podium to alert the orchestra that he was ready to begin. And then, to my horror, he began to conduct with his left arm only! His right arm hung limply at his side.

"Oh my God," I whispered to my friend standing next to me. "He is not moving his right arm!" I was afraid I had injured him in our session.

I waited, praying that he would begin using his right arm, the one I'd worked on. But he continued with his left, the orchestra nevertheless performing beautifully. Then, finally, he brought his right arm up and began using both arms. I heaved a sigh of relief. Both his arms moved with extraordinary grace and expressiveness. In that moment, the energy in the Shed suddenly shifted. The orchestra as well as the audience came alive. The change was palpable, literally sending ecstatic waves up my spine. The audience's excitement seemed to be similar to mine as the performance continued.

After the concert, I was walking back to my room when a car drove up beside me and the window rolled down. It was the conductor. He asked if I'd like a ride, and I accepted. As we drove to my place, I asked him how his right shoulder felt, and he said it was fine. It was feeling much better. I then explained that I'd been watching him conducting and had been concerned that he was having trouble with his right shoulder.

"Oh, not at all," he explained. "I became curious. I experimented to see if I could move my left arm with the same fluidity and ease I experienced with my right arm after my session with you."

"It looked like you were successful," I said.

"Yes. It certainly felt good to me," the conductor said.

Here was a man, one of the most esteemed orchestral conductors in the world, still seeking to learn and improve. He took the first opportunity to experiment with a new experience he had had and apply it to himself and his actions—and do this in front of a full orchestra and a huge audience. His learning switch was certainly on. His curiosity, his eagerness to learn, his willingness to take a risk, and his complete engagement in the process were all characteristics of the organic learner.

When we are engaged in this way, we often find that everything we encounter in our environment relates back to whatever we are working on, or trying to learn. A simple example of this is a story a friend told me about learning to ski. On and off the hill, she had experiences that related to what she was learning about balance and coordinating her physical responses as she was sliding down the hill on her skis. One day, while returning home from work on a bus, she noticed two boys skateboarding in a park. One older boy was very skillful, while a younger one was obviously just beginning to learn. Watching the contrast between the two boys, she saw something in the more skillful boy's movements that revealed how she could correct a movement she had been trying to master in her skiing. In that instant, she said, everything changed for her. She felt different in her body, and she could not wait for the weekend when she'd go skiing again so she could start practicing what she'd just witnessed.

One of the most colorful examples of how our brains work when our learning switch is on and we are engaged in organic learning is found in the story of Archimedes (ca. 287–212 BC), who is often credited with inventing geometry.

It is told that Archimedes was assigned the task of determining if a golden crown placed in his possession was truly made of gold or if it was a counterfeit. But he had to determine this without changing or damaging the very elaborately shaped crown. For several days, he puzzled over how this could be done. One day, he decided to take a bath. We can imagine him lowering himself into his bath and noticing that his body felt somewhat lighter, buoyed up by the water. He observed how some of the water displaced by his body flowed over the edge of the tub.

Suddenly, he had the solution to his problem—igniting an insight that we still use today in calculating the weight and density of an object. He realized that if he took a bar of gold that weighed exactly the same as the golden crown, both the crown and the bar should displace exactly the same amount of water. If the volume of water displaced by the crown was different from the volume displaced by the gold, it meant the crown was not pure gold. (For example, the density of gold is nearly twice that of lead.) The story goes that Archimedes was so excited by this discovery that he leaped from his bath and went running through the streets naked, shouting the news of his discovery.

This story shows the level of total involvement and the resulting high level of vitality we have when the learning switch is turned on and we engage in organic learning. We can imagine how Archimedes' brain became very active, perhaps with a virtual explosion of new activity. Remember in the previous chapter the image of each brain cell being a light? At the moment of his discovery, Archimedes' brain must have been ablaze.

The good news for us is that we don't have to be a genius mathematician like Archimedes or a famous orchestral conductor to experience this state of being. In fact, we have all experienced it in our childhoods and in other times in our lives. Perhaps it was with a sudden notion about a gift for a special person or a breakthrough moment at work. What we know about the brain and organic learning is that it is accompanied by increased activity and an outward movement to seek and create new information. It changes the way we experience our lives. Note in the story about Archimedes that the discovery that lit up his brain came about when he was involved in an activity that appeared to have little or no relationship to the problem he was attempting to solve. Archimedes had his insight about calculating weight and mass while getting into a tub to bathe! What made the big difference was his level of engagement, set into motion by the learning switch being turned on.

Exercise 3   Experience New Freedom of Movement

What you'll experience in this NeuroMovement exercise is that change comes about, whether it is reducing pain or improving our movements, not by forcing our bodies, but by "talking" to our brains. Improving how we move is a learning process. Remember, our brains tell our bodies how to move. If we're to change how we move, we have to provide our brains with new information. Without new information, our brains will just keep telling us the same old thing—and if that old information is resulting in pain or other limitation, we definitely want to change it. That's what *turning on the learning switch* is all about.

Preparation

Do this exercise in a place and at a time of day when you will be without interruptions for approximately ten minutes. Alternately, have a friend join you, with one of you reading the instructions while the other follows them. Wear comfortable, loose-fitting clothing and work with a straight-backed chair that allows you to have both feet comfortably on the floor. Work in your stocking feet so that you have good contact between your feet and the floor. Make sure you do all the movements easily, always within your comfort range—you don't want to strain your neck. The drawings will help guide you along.

THE EXERCISE

1. Sit on the edge of the chair with both feet flat on the floor and a comfortable distance apart. Approximately the width of your pelvis is ideal. Rest your hands, fingers down, on the tops of your thighs. Call this your neutral position. Turn your head to look to the right. Do so easily, always within your comfort range, without forcing anything, straining nothing. Take note of how far you turn your head. You might want to spot a visual reference point you can use to measure changes as you go along. Now turn your head to the left and find a similar reference point.

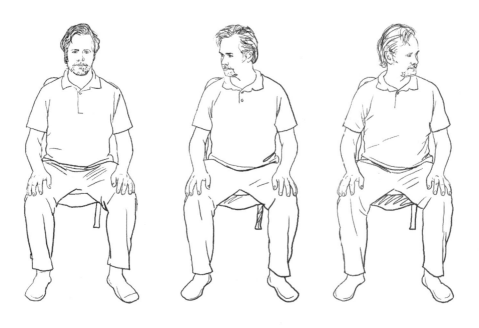

Note: In the rest of this lesson, I am only giving you instructions for the right side. But when you have finished the right side, you can simply do the left side by reversing right and left.

2. While still sitting on the edge of the chair, place your right hand a few inches behind you on the seat of the chair and lean back on it so it's bearing some of your weight. Turn your head to the right and then turn your head back to look straight ahead of you. Make sure you move easily within your comfortable range of motion and note how far to the right you see. Repeat this movement two or three times. Then come back to the middle, placing both your hands back on your thighs, stop, and rest for a moment.

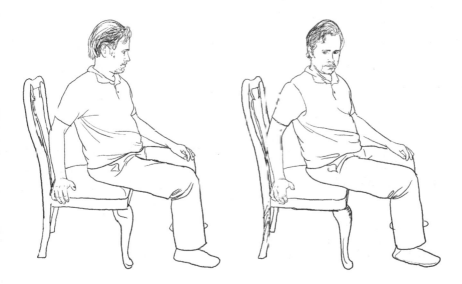

3. Again, sit on the edge of your chair and place your right hand behind you and lean on it as before. Now lift your left arm, bend your elbow, and rest your chin on the back of your hand. Gently turn your head and your arm together, as one unit, to the right and then come back to center. As you turn, make sure that your chin is in contact with the back of your left hand all the time. Do this

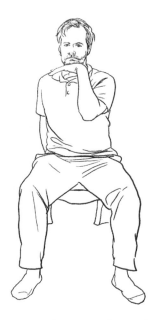
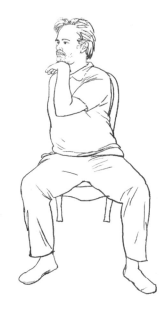

movement three or four times. Stop, come back to your neutral position, and rest for a moment. Notice if there are any changes in the way you are sitting or feeling.

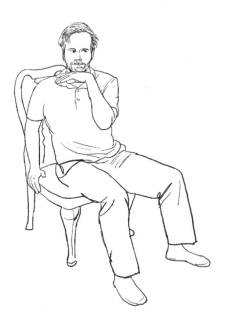

4. Using the same position as above, with your chin on the back of your left hand, turn to the right as far as is comfortable for you and hold that position. Now gently move only your eyes to the right and to the left. Repeat the movement three or four times, then stop and rest in your neutral position.

5. In the same position as step 4, turn as far as you can to the right comfortably and stay there. Now lift your left buttock off the chair an inch or so and put it back down three or four times. Feel how your ribs move on your left side, coming closer together and then moving farther apart as you lift and lower your left buttock. Stop, come back to neutral, and notice if you are sitting differently on your right buttock compared to the left.

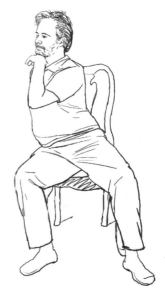

6. Once again, lean on your right hand behind you and turn your head to the right. Notice if your neck moves more easily and whether you see farther than before.

7. Now go back to your neutral position, with both hands palm down on the tops of your thighs. Gently turn your head to the right, then to the left, and notice whether you turn your head more easily to the right than to the left. You have just experienced the power of turning on your learning switch.

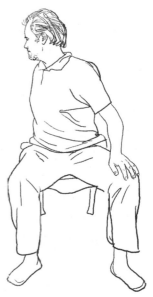

You may do this exercise on the other side; however, before you do, for at least an hour or so, let yourself experience the differences between your right side and your left side as you move and go about your life.

TURNOFFS AND TURN-ONS

You might be asking, "If we come into life with our learning switch turned on, and organic learning is our natural state, what turns the switch off?" It would certainly seem logical, especially since our vitality depends so much on it, that we would do everything in our power to keep it turned on. But the human experience is more complicated than that. While our brains contain all the functions needed to create high levels of vitality, they also possess the potential for reducing our vitality, even to the point that we feel like emotionless robots.

As highly evolved as we might like to think we humans are, the old reptilian part of our brains still influences much of our behavior. It is this part of the brain that triggers the so-called fight-or-flight response. Researchers now tell us that whenever we are confronted with a perceived threat, our old reptilian brain sends out signals to the rest of our brain, and thus out to our body, that cause us to want to do one of two things: fight or run. And if we can't do either of those, we freeze; we essentially "play possum" until the danger passes. This is a survival tactic. Whether we fight, flee, or freeze, what eludes us at that moment is the ability to explore and discover alternate ways to resolve the challenge. Out of those three possible responses, we most often choose the freeze mode and inhibit, or repress, our impulse to fight or flee.

In Sigmund Freud's *Civilization and Its Discontents,* he made a case for the fact that repression—a shutting down of sensory input, as well as erotic and aggressive feelings—is an inevitable offshoot of civilization's demands on us. To put it in the terms of this chapter, we get very good at freezing, which means that we turn off the learning switch. After all, if you're angry at your boss or a coworker, it's not usually acceptable to start a fight. And if you run, the chances are you won't have a job the next day. Similarly, if your fight-or-flight response is triggered by a family member, you may fight, you may even run, but most of us have learned there are serious consequences if we go too far with either of these; freezing is the most socially acceptable thing to do.

The cost of freezing is very high. Our vitality disappears. Not only do our feelings begin to numb, but we also start tuning out our responses to other stimuli. Our response is often "Okay, I'll just shut up, do what I'm told to do, and nothing more" or we are simply too fearful to explore, discover, and invent. This is anything but an organic-learning state.

Generally, our struggles with the fight-flight-freeze experience is labeled "stress." Anyone who has ever had this kind of experience—and who hasn't?—knows how uncomfortable it is. Our pelvis, back, shoulder, and fist muscles may go into a state of chronic tension; we may have elevated heart and breathing rates; we may develop digestive problems; some people may feel light-headed, depressed, and distracted. As stress builds, such symptoms become increasingly uncomfortable, even unbearably painful, leading to disease. At this point, we may be labeled as needing to take time off from work or home responsibilities; we sign up for stress-management classes, or we medicate ourselves to take away the pain.

There are times when a vacation, a massage, a class in stress management, or even medication can be a godsend. Given the pressures of life, we shouldn't pass judgment on any of these. However, we should not turn a blind eye to the price we pay in terms of lost vitality for indulging only in these ways of handling stress. Groundbreaking research by Fulbright scholar Angela Patmore, described in her book *The Truth About Stress,* suggests that how we handle stress in our lives can either empower us or tranquilize us. In an interview in *Ode* magazine (May 2007), Patmore explains that by calming people down as a form of stress management, you "reduce their coping skills, making people more cowardly and unwilling to take up new challenges, through which they can grow in life."

If handled well, Patmore asserts, we expand our repertoire of skills and information; we meet life's difficulties with the confidence of knowing we have the inner resources to do so successfully. Best-selling author-educator Ronald Gross, a leading expert on lifelong learning, points out that our brains thrive on challenge and flow. Gross explains that we need to find that optimal state of embracing our challenges, of finding that place where our brains are stretched, but we can do it, if we give it our all. The result, Gross says, "is 'flow'—that wonderful state where time seems to pass swiftly, and we are exhilarated by the sense of accomplishment." This is an example of how turning on the learning switch and gaining the vitality we long to have is really a choice.

Let's be reminded here of the profound link between brain activity, the creation of new possibilities and experiences, and our level of vitality. If we want to be vital, we need to bring increasing attention to organic learning, realizing that anything we do—be it in the realm of academic learning, skill acquisition, or self-exploration—can be approached in this way, that is, with the learning switch on. The good news is that turning on the learning switch is a skill we can develop.

EXERCISE 4   WHAT TURNS OFF YOUR LEARNING SWITCH

It is useful to discover how and where you tend to turn off the learning switch. With this knowledge, you can turn the switch back on, or avoid turning it off in the first place. Some of the common turnoffs I have observed with myself, my students, and my clients over the years are feeling rushed; assuming there is only one way of doing something; trying to learn by rote or by a set formula; believing yourself to be inadequate, perhaps because you had been told you were stupid or inept in some area; blaming—either oneself or others; personal defensiveness; and any areas of past trauma, neglect, or abuse that undermine self-trust or the ability to take in new information. What are some of your learning-switch turnoffs? Identify an area in your life you want to bring more vitality to. It could be your social life, your physical fitness, your professional life, even your health. Ask yourself if you have been doing any learning in that area lately. Most likely, the answer will be no. Try to identify any beliefs, or past experiences, that have turned off your learning switch. Fear, blame, shame, someone else's negative opinion, and past failures are very common learning-switch turnoffs. The good news is that your brain is always at the ready to turn on the learning switch. All you have to do, once you have identified where you want to turn the switch back on, is to choose to resume learning through classes, reading, your own exploration and experimentation, or any other means.

THE ABCs OF TURNING ON YOUR LEARNING SWITCH

We've all experienced what it's like to have the learning switch turned on and to be immersed in organic learning. Perhaps you can remember it from childhood, when each day brought a seemingly endless flow of new experiences and your brain was busy creating new information that would become an integral part of your life. You may also recall times when you were excitedly engaged in learning something new that was very near and dear to your heart; this strong sense of emotional involvement in the learning is indicative of the learning switch being turned on. Maybe you've noticed that during our discussions of the learning switch and organic learning, your memories of those past experiences were awakened and you were able to feel the excitement and high levels of vitality you enjoyed during those times.

Simply reading about organic learning and the learning switch, and having your own memories of these experiences stirred up, can help you start turning on your learning switch. Beyond that, you can develop skills to turn it on at will. Once you have developed the ability to turn on the learning switch at will, you have gained a skill for restoring and maintaining vitality throughout your life. Remember, living with the learning switch turned on is a way of being, one that provides you with all the benefits of living with vitality.

As you begin the process of learning how to turn on your learning switch voluntarily, keep in mind that just as in learning to ride a bicycle, communicate well with your spouse, ski, or develop any other skill, daily practice strengthens your abilities. In the beginning, plan to spend five to ten minutes each day to do the following steps, alone or with others:

FIVE STEPS TO TURNING ON THE LEARNING SWITCH TO EXPERIENCE A VITAL AND EXCITING NEW LIFE

1. KNOW THAT IT IS POSSIBLE FOR YOU TO TURN ON THE LEARNING SWITCH YOURSELF. Begin with the understanding that *it can be done;* you can turn on the learning switch and make organic learning, with all its attendant gains in vitality, a part of your everyday life. If doubts arise, remember the lessons of the true pioneers of history who were surrounded by naysayers, yet who prevailed. Roger Bannister, the man who, in 1954, broke the four-minute mile, was surrounded by scientists "proving" the human body was not capable of breaking the four-minute mile. Bannister not only did it, but since that time hundreds of other runners have done the same; in fact, there are now high school runners who better Bannister's record. Turning on the learning switch is nowhere near that kind of challenge the four-minute mile was, since organic learning is a natural part of life. Still, knowing with total assurance that you can make organic learning a part of your everyday life is an important first step in your success.

2. CREATE AN IMAGINARY PLACE IN YOUR MIND WHERE THE LEARNING SWITCH GETS TURNED ON AND ORGANIC LEARN-

ING OCCURS. Think of your mind as having many rooms. Most of these rooms are occupied with your habitual stream of thoughts and feelings. These rooms are sometimes filled to overflowing with things to do, things to remember, ideas and beliefs that repeat themselves, and feelings we have about people and activities in our lives. Then imagine there is one room in which the lights turn on any time you step into it. Once you are in that room, you immediately become curious. You discover the new in the daily and mundane. You experience yourself and the people around you in new ways, and your mind fills up with new ideas. First, create this illuminated room vividly in your mind, so that you will be able to quickly get a mental picture of it, and feel yourself in it, any time you wish. Furnish your imaginary room. Decide on the colors of the walls, the texture of the floor, and the objects you want to have in this room. Don't forget windows if you'd like to have a view— even the view outside can be important. Once this imaginary room is well established in your mind, choose a situation from your everyday life that you can bring into this space. You might also want to bring your image of this room into your mind when you want to discover the new and bring change and improvement to an ongoing situation or activity. Imagine yourself in this room when you are talking with another person, doing a yoga exercise, playing golf, participating in a business meeting, or even standing in line at the supermarket. As you become increasingly familiar with how it feels to have your learning switch on, recalling your image of this room will instantly transport you into the organic-learning frame of mind.

3. BECOME INTENTIONAL. Choose an area in your life that is important to you personally and that you can feel safe exploring with your learning switch turned on. This might have to do with looking at the quality of your interactions with your child, the way you write memos at work, your beliefs about having money, how you do a daily walk or run, or any of a seemingly infinite number of issues that arise in our lives. Begin by setting the intention that

you want to have the learning switch on as you visit the subject you have chosen. Do this with the intention that you are not going to try to accomplish a specific outcome, such as communicating more peacefully with your child, walking faster or farther, writing more concise memos, or whatever is applicable. Be aware that this intention is different from a goal. Intention is an action, something you do right now. Just have the intention that you will notice and experience the new; you will expect the unexpected, and discover what you haven't seen or noticed before, or something you couldn't have dreamed possible. You might notice your habitual "stories" trying to jump in, such as thinking that what you are doing is ridiculous or getting caught up in an argument you never resolved with your child, or with your own interpretations of something that has happened in the past. When stories such as these arise, say to yourself, "Thank you for sharing." Observe yourself noting the old stories, then letting them go and finally re-creating your intent, untainted by your own or anyone else's stories, interpretations, or analyses. If you feel yourself applying old patterns of thoughts and feelings, just note that you are doing that and allow them to pass through your mind.

I'm reminded of a story that was told to me many years ago by my teacher about D'Arcy Thompson, a famous British biologist. As a young student, D'Arcy's life was changed when his professor sat him down in a room in front of a desk that held only a tortoise shell. D'Arcy was told to look at this shell to see what he might discover. A bit confused but willing to comply, he sat for hours looking at the shell and seeing only a shell. One day passed, then two. Nothing happened. He was ready to give up and go home. Then, on the eighth day, he saw what no one had ever seen before. He suddenly had an insight that the growth and form of all living things complied with physical laws and mechanics, adding a whole new dimension to the study of evolution. Nobel laureate Peter Medawar called D'Arcy's book *On Growth and Form* "the finest work of literature in all the annals of science. . . ." D'Arcy's work is a prime example of organic learning, which was triggered when he focused his intentionality on the discovery of the new and unexpected.

We learn from his experience that regardless of the object or issue we are focusing on, we discover the new not by *trying* to learn, and not through our efforts to make sense of our discoveries, but by allowing our brains to do their work, without limiting how they will use this new information. Einstein spoke of something he called "recombinant play," which simply meant that one allowed information to mix all together like in a wonderful stew where flavors mingle, find their own connections, and produce something one could never have predicted.

Drop all inclinations to judge right or wrong, good or bad; let go of any attachments you might have with a desire to *do something* about what you are taking in. Just hold your intention with curiosity, interest, and nonjudgment. This might be difficult at first, but the more you practice this process, even for a few minutes a day, the more you will begin to see changes in yourself, letting go of routines and habits and ultimately experiencing not only more and greater vitality, but a life that gets increasingly more thrilling as time passes.

If you are bringing this process to a relationship with a family member, a coworker, or a friend, hold the intention that you will be seeking new information out of which will come a fresh new way of relating to that person. Soon you will begin to feel a subtle shift. The first signs of this will be a quiet excitement—indeed, a new sense of vitality.

You might also bring this process with you during a walk in nature. As you notice the wildflowers, perhaps their color will seem brighter, their scent stronger, their very existence more miraculous than ever before. You might notice shapes that you have never seen before. The air might seem more fragrant, and its movement on your skin more pleasurable. The first signs of a transformation occurring in a relationship will be that you feel excited by perceiving something new that you had not previously noticed about the other person. You may feel you are discovering a whole new side of him or her, one you never guessed was possible and at the same time you might discover new sides to you. All of these are signs of the learning switch turning on and your stepping into the light of organic learning.

4. GET CURIOUS ABOUT YOURSELF. No matter what you are doing, whether consciously learning a new skill, recreational activity, academic subject, or anything else, make it *personal* by paying attention to how what you are learning is affecting you emotionally, physically, intellectually, or even spiritually. Let's say you are learning ballroom dancing. Notice how it is affecting the way your body feels: Maybe you feel more flexible, more expansive, lighter, and more sensual. If you are learning a new language, see if you can find a pen pal for whom that language is their native tongue. Nowadays, many movie DVDs allow you to select different languages, either dubbed or in subtitles; select a favorite movie of yours, one for which you have felt some emotional involvement, and watch it in that language. When you read a book or watch a movie or a TV show, ask yourself why you are attracted to certain characters. What is it in you that is stimulated by that person? Maybe a character on a TV show impresses you because of her leadership skills; acknowledge this to yourself, and ask how you might bring your experience of that character into your everyday life. Or maybe you read a novel in which a character changed something about herself that improved her relationship with her spouse. Get curious and try doing something like that in your own relationship. Know that everything you are thinking, feeling, and seeing in these moments when your learning switch is turned on is in the service of you. They are your discoveries, and only need to be meaningful and important to you.

5. RECOGNIZE YOUR OWN GROWING LEADERSHIP. Pay particular attention to the ways you are taking an increasingly greater leadership role in how you experience your life. Turning on the learning switch and unleashing the vitality that comes with it does not happen by itself. It is a choice that we make. Children are exceptionally vital and energetic because they are intensely immersed in organic learning all the time. However, for them the process is spontaneous by virtue of their youth and innocence. When we, as adults, take the kind of leadership role I'm describing, choosing our own process of learning, we are empowered; we have endless resources of energy, and we are inspired.

As you notice yourself gaining the skill of turning on your learning switch and doing so by choice, you may also feel a sense of lightness, freedom, and greater power, and a new appreciation for who you are and what you bring. Your newfound skill of turning on your learning switch will be like opening a new door and crossing into a brand-new territory—a transformative experience that will light up millions of new cells in your brain, and fill you with newfound vitality.

EXERCISE 5 TURNING ON THE LEARNING SWITCH

WHAT'S YOUR VITALITY QUOTIENT?

On a scale of 1 to 5, rate yourself on each of the following statements, with 5 being always, 3 being occasionally, 1 being never.

1. Whether at home or at work, I easily make any task interesting or pleasurable.

2. I often find myself interested in new ideas about myself or how things work—when watching TV or a movie, engaging in a conversation, surfing the Internet, or reading.

3. I discover new things when visiting familiar places, whether it's my own hometown or another country I've previously visited.

4. When exercising, I experiment with and frequently find ways to improve how I do my routines.

5. I enjoy exploring and discovering new ways of communicating with those around me.

6. I welcome opinions different from mine because I find it interesting and enjoyable to expand my knowledge and beliefs.

7. In my sexual relationship, I am interested in finding new ways to mutually share deeper connection and intimacy.

Score Yourself
24–35 points = high
15–23 points = medium
1–14 points = low

Go through the seven statements above and choose the ones on which you scored the lowest. Take some time to think about ways to improve your scores in those areas. The statements themselves will guide you.

Three

Subtlety—Experience the Power of Gentleness

Deeper and more profound,
The door of all subtleties!
—Lao-tzu

In Eckhart Tolle's international bestseller *The Power of Now*, he observes that "dangerous activities such as car racing and mountain climbing" force those who participate in them to be *in the now* they must pay close attention and notice subtle differences between one moment and the next. If they fail to notice these differences, and fail to respond effectively, it can be disastrous for them. When we are living this way, acutely sensitive to the subtleties of each moment, we are in what Tolle describes as an "intensely alive state." We are highly attuned to the feeling of what happens.

We are often fascinated by people who engage in extreme sports or other forms of heroic activities, which is why they are so often the subjects of movies and literature. They are charismatic, tremendously alive—vital! They are able to respond and act creatively and effectively at any moment, especially in moments of great need. We remember them because they come to represent what it means to live life fully. This also happens to be the classic description of the *warrior* mentality, a way of being present and available, responsive in highly effective ways to all that life might bring us, however we may have chosen to live it.

We admire these heroes and warriors because we recognize ourselves in them. Deep inside, a part of us knows we could be like them. Psychologists tell us that we cannot admire a quality or potential in others that we don't have in ourselves. Think about it the next time you are watching a movie or hear a story that inspires you. See if you can capture moments from your own life when you acted in a similar way. Chances are that you'll remember at least one time when you experienced yourself functioning in an optimal way, fully in the present and highly attuned to whatever was happening, however briefly. For most of us, this will be in activities less dramatic than piloting a racecar around a track at two hundred miles per hour. What's relevant here is not the event itself but the quality of your experience; that is, how fully engaged you were.

For our purposes with Subtlety and NeuroMovement, it is useful to look at ways of being in the now in your everyday activities, and experiencing the vitality that comes with a normal day in your life. You certainly don't have to take up bungee jumping, parachuting from airplanes, or some other extreme sport to experience this intensely alive state. On the contrary, the human brain—body, mind, and spirit—are put together in such a way that you can create this heightened vitality any time you wish.

MINIMIZE FORCE TO MAXIMIZE ATTUNEMENT

There is a key aspect of the warrior—of being attuned to what is happening—that often gets overlooked, and that is *elegance*. Elegance depends on our being able to feel what is going on for us, both in the outside world and within us. We can see this elegance in a good martial artist who effortlessly performs a difficult and powerful feat; or in a leader who inspires us with just a few words; or in a dancer who seems to fly like a bird; or in an artist, such as Picasso, who could draw one continuous line on a piece of paper and create the image of a lovely woman. This elegance is at the heart of our dance with life—it is where we experience vitality firsthand.

In contrast to the elegance of the warrior, a friend recently shared a story about a woman he hired to clean his home once a week. He had purchased all the best equipment, including a top-of-the-line vacuum cleaner, to make her work easier and to ensure the best job. Every day she came to do the vacuuming, however, he noticed that she worked herself into a sweat. She yanked the vacuum cleaner back and forth in fast, jerky motions, sometimes slamming it into the walls or the furniture, until the casing of the machine was badly bruised, to say nothing of the beating the furniture had taken. He could not understand why she was vacuuming so forcefully or why she seemed not to notice the wake of destruction she was leaving behind. She was using so much force and vigor moving around the vacuum cleaner that it actually was not working as efficiently as it was designed to do. The woman was so excessively forceful in her vacuuming that he feared she would ruin the carpet, the furniture, and the machine—and very possibly produce an injury to her own body!

This is the perfect example of how excessive force, at the very least, drains our energy and taxes our systems, increasing difficulty as well as causing injury, distress, and even illness. Excessive use of force, be it physical, mental, emotional, or spiritual, blunts our vitality; it makes us less able to feel, to fully experience what it means to be attuned to whatever we are engaged in. In addition, we get aches and pains, experience limitation and suffering, and at the end of the day feel older than need be. When we reduce force, we become more fully present; we become more sensitive to what we're doing, and we begin to notice finer differences.

Through the essential I call Subtlety, we're able to respond in an elegant way to what is happening both inside and outside ourselves and to make subtle adjustments in the ways we use our bodies and minds, to achieve whatever we wish to achieve with a minimum of effort.

I am here reminded of a challenge faced by NASA some years ago. The astronauts discovered that the gloves they had to wear in space were so thick that it was difficult for them to feel small objects or perform many of the delicate movements required of them. They were unable to feel subtle differences. A scientist and rehabilitation physician by the name of Paul Bach-y-Rita solved the astronauts' problem by adding electronic sensors to the gloves that transmitted signals from them to the astronauts' hands. In this way, the astronauts gained "sensitivity" that allowed them to feel subtle differences and make the very fine and precise movements required of them.

When we reduce force, it is like what happens for the astronauts when they put on their special "feeling" gloves: We immediately gain the ability to feel subtler and subtler differences. The advantage we have over the astronauts is that we don't require external paraphernalia to gain this sensitivity. Thanks to the power of our brains, we just need to reduce the force.

EXERCISE 1   WORK SMARTER, NOT HARDER

As you are learning in this chapter, reducing force increases your ability to feel, thus bringing you into the present and waking up your brain so that you can find new solutions. By reducing force and increasing your ability to feel subtle differences, you give your brain access to new information that allows it to upgrade the organization and quality of whatever you are doing. The improved organization allows you to live more efficiently, effectively, and creatively. You get things done with increased pleasure, and have more energy left at the end of the day.

PREPARATION

Set aside ten or fifteen minutes when you will not be interrupted by another person, the phone, the TV, or any other distractions. It is best to do this exercise with a mat on the floor or on a firm, flat surface large enough to do all of the movements comfortably and freely.

INSTRUCTIONS

You may have noticed that whenever you experience limitation in your movements, your first reaction is to try to force your body past the limitation, often through "stretching." The following exercise allows you to experience what it's like to move beyond limitations not by forcing or stretching but by *decreasing* the force.

1. Lie down on your back on your mat or other comfortable but firm, flat surface.

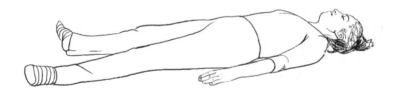

2. Raise your knees, drawing your feet toward your buttocks. Have the soles of your feet standing flat on the mat and approximately a foot apart.

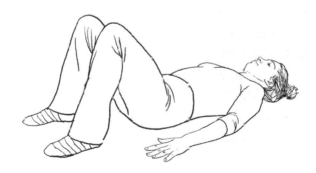

3. Cross your right leg over your left.

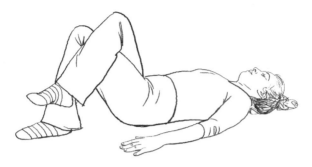

4. Gently tilt your legs, still crossed, to the right. Without forcing them in any way, let the weight of your legs bring them closer to the floor on your right. Then come back to center. Do this movement three or four times and feel how far down toward the floor your crossed legs will go without any forcing whatsoever.

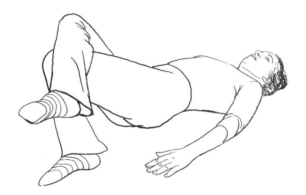

5. With your legs in the same position as in step 4, attempt to force (stretch) your legs to go lower than before, but make sure you don't hurt yourself. Do this—stretching—once or twice. Then go back to center and allow your crossed legs to go down without forcing them in any way. Do you notice any improvement? Most likely not. Make sure for the remainder of this exercise to do the movements as gently as you can. Move only as far as it is truly comfortable and easy for you. As you continue, notice if this approach results in more noticeable changes than those you felt by forcing your body.

6. Uncross your legs, lengthen them out on the floor, and rest for a moment.

7. Now lift both your knees and place your feet in the position you had them in step 2. Interlace your fingers and place your hands behind your head. Begin to lift your head with the help of your hands—the elbows come closer to each other—and then lower your head and hands back to the floor and let the elbows open back to the sides. Make sure to lift your head only as high as it is comfortable for you to do. That means you might lift your head only a couple of inches. These are not crunches. Do this *very gently* four or five times. Can you begin to feel your ribs moving? More softness in your chest?

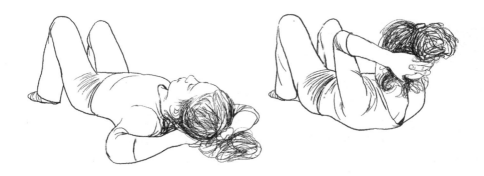

8. Rest for a moment, and feel any changes in the way you're lying on the floor.

9. Bend your legs, cross your right leg over the left, interlace your fingers behind your head, and then comfortably (without forcing) tilt your knees to the right. Stay with the knees tilted to the right, and then lift and lower your head as before, using your hands and arms to do the lifting. Make sure to let your hands and head rest on the floor for a second or two before lifting the head again. Do this *very gently* four or five times. Stop, uncross your legs, and rest for a moment.

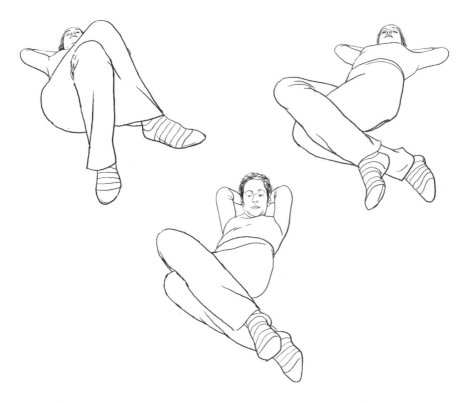

10. When you feel you are ready, cross your right knee over the left as before and simply tilt your knees to the right. Are your legs going down a bit lower? At the same time, is it actually easier to do?

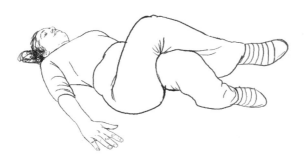

11. Rest and check out how you are feeling. Does your right leg feel different from the left? Does it feel longer? Lighter?

12. You may now do this whole sequence for your left side.

PARADOX: INCREASE YOUR POWER BY REDUCING FORCE

As strange as it might seem, there's a little of the woman with the vacuum cleaner in each of us. And no wonder. Most of us have grown up with slogans such as "No pain, no gain," and "You have to try harder if you want to succeed." The idea of trying harder and using more force is conditioned into every cell of our being. In addition, we have experienced some successes by trying harder, and these successes reinforce anything we've been told about it. You probably can't remember back to the earliest events in your life, but you've probably seen a small child doing pre-school jigsaw puzzles for the first time. In the beginning, she can't make the pieces fit, so she intensifies her efforts, pressing them as hard as she can into the puzzle frame; at last, she is successful. The pieces miraculously fit.

"Hey, using force really works!" the child thinks, victorious with her accomplishment.

What she couldn't have known at that moment, of course, is that she found the right fit by luck. If anything, reduction of force would have made it much easier for her to notice what she was doing and orient the shapes of the puzzle pieces to one another. We all, of course, begin in this place as children, but as we evolve, we develop in our refinement and learn to reduce force, become more attuned with the present, and accomplish fine motor movements like this easily. In the meantime, the little girl's brain registered her experience that force seemed to get her what she wanted. She learns this lesson—that force made the puzzle piece fit—early on and carries it with her until she finds some reason to amend it.

The use of excessive force often appears to get us what we want in adulthood, as well as in childhood. It takes us a while to discover that, if anything, we succeed despite excessive force. Old habits and perceptions then carry over into adulthood. When we set out to accomplish something, we tend to do what the child does, especially if we are not sure we can do it. We tend to apply excessive physical, emotional, and mental force. We clench our teeth, hold our breath, and make funny faces when trying to remove the tight lid from a jar. We raise our voices and talk faster as we try to give road directions to a person who doesn't know our language well. We get more and more emotional and loud when arguing with a loved one, as if by doing so we might break through the impasse we are experiencing.

But what does all of this have to do with vitality and NeuroMovement? The answers may surprise you. As we reduce excessive force, and use only as much as required, we become attuned to what we are doing at that moment. We experience whatever we are doing in a more sensual way; we feel more when we touch. We hear things we didn't hear when we were *efforting* so much. We see finer differences, and colors appear more vibrant. We feel our bodies, our muscles and bones, more fully. As we reduce force, we come into the present, and awaken our vitality.

EXERCISE 2   HAVE EYES AND SEE, EARS AND HEAR, HEART AND FEEL

Think of a person in your life with whom you have recurring difficulty, with some emotional intensity on your part. It might be with your child about his or her homework. It might be with your spouse about helping with housework, or any particular difficulty you have with a friend, or a colleague at work. Create in your imagination the challenging situation you have with that person and let yourself feel the emotions that you usually experience in that situation. Then reduce the intensity of these emotions—remembering that it is all in your imagination. Pause, and let yourself experience this feeling of lowered intensity. Now deliberately increase the intensity of your emotions, perhaps even exaggerating what you usually experience with that person. Pause and experience that feeling for a moment. Then reduce the intensity again. Repeat this emotional movement of increasing and decreasing intensity four or five times.

Now that you have done this mental rehearsal as described above, you are ready to apply it in real life. When you do, you will notice that two things begin to occur: As you reduce your emotional intensity, you will be able to become more attuned to the other person and better able to hear what he or she is trying to say. You will be more alert and vital, able to come up with new ideas, feelings, behaviors, and solutions. What you are also likely to find is that the other person will feel more at ease and less defensive in your presence. Subtlety literally brings people closer.

NOTICING SUBTLE DIFFERENCES

The correlation between discerning subtle differences, being *in the now,* and vitality is impossible to deny. Our sense of vitality is closely associated with our brain's ability to perceive differences, and it is through this perception of differences, an important part of NeuroMovement, that our brains create new information. Sometimes just a shift of our attention in the direction of noticing subtle differences can be transformational, awakening us to our own vitality in surprising, unexpected ways. Do you remember the image in previous chapters of our brain cells *lighting up?* This happens when our brains perceive differences in the stimuli that are coming in and begin creating something new. When most of the stimulation the brain receives is the same, or perceived as the same, we simply don't notice it and the brain can't respond to it, nor do anything new with it. In Eckhart Tolle's observation about mountain climbers and racecar drivers, the more extreme the danger the participants are in, the more they need to notice the subtlest of differences, or they certainly won't be doing what they are doing for very long. They are required to develop their ability to notice subtle differences and then operate in such a way that they are attuned to the smallest changes—changes that you or I might overlook.

In our everyday lives, it's easy to lull ourselves into a place of complacency and familiarity, sticking pretty close to daily routines in our lives, at work, at home, and at play. Eventually, even though there is always change and variation in our lives, our activities are similar enough that our brains don't particularly notice those variations. Remember Hebbian plasticity from the previous chapter? Once we have formed successful patterns, the more we use them, the more deeply ingrained they become. Even when the stimulus changes over time, our brains tend to perceive it as the same. We go along as if one moment were pretty much like another, without creating anything that we would perceive as new.

To achieve vitality, we must awaken ourselves to subtle differences. As I was writing one afternoon, I gazed out the window briefly and saw a middle-aged couple walking down the street. I had seen the woman before. She walked past our home about the same time every day. But I had never seen the man before. I became aware of the difference between the woman's gait and the man's. She walked elegantly, with ease, obviously enjoying what she was doing. He, by contrast, walked very stiffly, as if each step required tremendous effort.

At the place where the walkway is interrupted by our driveway, the surface of the sidewalk tips slightly downhill and to the left. When the man came to this area, he suddenly stumbled against the woman and would have fallen had she not responded quickly to steady him.

At that moment, I saw a living example of the very thing I was writing about. I speculated that the man, who was putting a great deal of effort and force into his walking, probably spent most of his time indoors where floors were flat, smooth, predictable surfaces. With little new information about walking, with few new challenges presented day after day, his brain had had few opportunities to create anything new and he gradually became more rigid. Because walking down the street was different from his usual everyday activity of moving around on level floors, the man responded by putting more effort (force) into what he was doing. This is a common response for most of us when we are presented with something we find difficult for us. When we find ourselves in a new situation, our automatic tendency is to use more force than necessary to do whatever it is that we are doing. By exerting great effort as he walked down the street, the man desensitized himself to the changes in the surface of the ground. Even though the stimuli from his feet stepping on to the changing ground were coming to his brain, they were not strong enough to be noticed over the great effort he was making while walking. As a result, his brain didn't perceive the change in the curb and was unable to respond appropriately, so he stumbled.

When the man came to the driveway where the sidewalk tipped, his brain continued to do what it had been doing every day indoors. It didn't have the information to respond in a quick, elegant, or appropriate way. No matter how much effort the man put into walking across the driveway area, his brain couldn't make use of all the stimulation that was coming his way because he was unable to perceive the differences.

The woman, who was enjoying the walk, negotiated the hill and the surface of the driveway easily. Even when the man stumbled, she was able to respond quickly and put her arm out to help him steady himself.

As I watched them move past my house and down the street, I noted that while the two of them were approximately the same age—probably a married couple—the woman's responsiveness and wakefulness to what was going on was much greater than the man's. Her movements were far more flexible, confident, and strong than her partner's. To my surprise, soon after rescuing the man from falling, she stopped to smell the roses in front of my house, then gestured enthusiastically as if to tell the man how wonderful the flowers were. She obviously not only noticed the roses, but also wasn't going to miss the opportunity to enjoy them. The man, by contrast, seemed uncomfortable—if not a little irritated—by the whole thing.

The experience was a task for him. Not only was he stiff in his body, but he also waited somewhat impatiently as the woman stopped to admire the gardens along the way, unable to join her in her enthusiasm.

Which of these two was the more vital and alive? Which of them was more able to "be in the now," as Tolle might have described it? Obviously, it was the woman, who responded easily and spontaneously to unexpected change. We might even say that for her the walk was a peak experience, while for the man the walk was a challenge, requiring a great deal of effort.

Gain Without Strain

Let's take the above example a bit further. While the following story is about a different man who was a client of mine—I'll call him Gary—it could just as well have been about the man I saw walking by my house that day. Gary and his wife had decided that they wanted to spend more leisure time together. They thought it would be nice to do this by getting a little exercise each morning and enjoying the neighborhood. Gary, who was a civil engineer for a large architectural firm, had been having a little back pain and had remarked to his wife, Alyssa, that he was feeling old, stiff, and lethargic at the end of the day. He'd been athletic in his twenties and thirties, and now, entering his forties, he didn't like what he was experiencing. He really wanted to change.

His doctor gave him a clean bill of health but recommended that he get more exercise. In the beginning, like most of us, Gary put way too much force into what he was doing. To get himself in shape, he started weight lifting, climbing steeper hills, and taking much longer walks than he and his wife had been taking. After all, when he'd played football in high school, that's what they did to get in condition for the season. Not realizing that it was his brain as much as his body that needed the workout, he used excessive force in his new regimen. Not only was he overriding pain messages that were telling him he was harming himself, but his excessive efforts also made it impossible for his brain to perceive subtleties; the result was that his brain did not have the information required to redirect his body in ways that would better match what he was trying to do. And so, the more effort he put into these workouts, the more tight and rigid he became, and his back pain and stiffness worsened. Feeling less vital than ever, he feared that what he was experiencing was the result of aging—which he would soon learn was not the case. That's when he was referred to me by a friend of his.

After hearing his story and examining how he was standing, sitting, and walking, I told Gary that he would need to cut way back on his exercise. Instead of lifting the heaviest weights he possibly could, I asked that he lift very light weights for a while—and not climb more steep hills for a few weeks. He looked at me as if I were a madwoman. I told him I wanted him to find a nice level place where he could walk in a leisurely way with his wife while enjoying their surroundings. I suggested a beautiful woodsy park not far from their home.

He tried to argue that what he'd learned when he was younger was that you had to go through a little pain to get any improvement in strength and flexibility. I told him I understood that this was what many people believed but that actually the opposite was true. I guaranteed that if he followed my suggestions, he would be lifting heavier weights and walking farther within a few weeks. In addition, he would be enjoying greater energy and feeling more flexible and confident, and his back pain would begin vanishing in a few days.

Gary came in for two more appointments with me, during which time I had him do some very simple floor exercises. Through these exercises, I guided and encouraged him to reduce the force with which he moved. He discovered that when he did this, his body moved much better, with greater ease and pleasure.

At first, when he bent down to touch his toes, he was only able to get halfway down. When he bounced harder in an effort to reach his toes, I quickly stopped him and had him greatly reduce the force. As he reduced the force, he was able to feel what he was doing, and soon his hands were two-thirds of the way down toward his feet. For Gary, changing his attitude and beliefs about needing to force and try harder was as challenging, if not more challenging, than changing how he was doing his exercises. In one week, he was noticing a change in his body. He was feeling great during his walks. He and his wife had already effortlessly doubled the distance they went each morning.

Gary continued lifting lighter weights as part of his new regimen. Doing so gave him a chance to feel how to use his back in a better way. He began increasing the weights in tiny increments so that he wasn't feeling any additional stress on his body. I asked him if he was noticing any change in his back pain. He enthusiastically reported that the pain and stiffness were gone and that at the end of the day he had so much energy that he was getting things done around the house that he'd been putting off for years. He reported that he was not only feeling more energetic and flexible, but that he was also feeling younger and more vital than he'd felt in over a decade.

BREAKING THE VICIOUS CIRCLE

The changes Gary experienced of increased strength, flexibility, and vitality came about when he reduced force in his exercises. More than a century ago, a psychophysiologist by the name of Ernst Heinrich Weber showed that our sensitivity to a stimulus diminishes as the background intensity of that stimulus increases. To demonstrate this, you might pick up and hold a two-pound book; holding the book represents the *background effort* your muscles are exerting. Think of the weight of the book as the background stimulus. Then, let's say, you place a half-ounce pen on top of the book. The sensations coming from your muscles and joints as you hold the book are too strong for you to notice the increased weight of the pen. Your brain cannot perceive the difference. But put down the book and hold instead a one-ounce letter in your hand; place the same pen on top of the letter, and your brain will certainly notice it. Here's how this principle applies to Gary's exercise regimen.

When Gary exercised with excessive effort, he could not feel what was going on with his body at a subtle enough level. As a result, he was confined to repeating his existing patterns that were at the root of his pain, limitation, and fatigue. If he had been able to feel more, he could have better matched what his body was doing to the task of lifting the weights or walking up and down the hills. Before Gary learned to reduce the force while exercising and to feel more, pain was the only signal he recognized as a stopping point. After he learned to move with less effort, he recognized more subtle signals that guided him how to change what he was doing so that he stopped getting the pain altogether. Noticing more subtle differences allowed Gary's brain to organize his movements in more efficient ways that left him energized, feeling positive about himself and his life. Through NeuroMovement he experienced more vitality and enjoyed himself in the present.

When he exercised with excessive force, he ended up with minor injuries and muscular soreness that comes with overexertion. As he was quick to admit himself, he wasn't finding much pleasure in the workouts themselves, mostly because he was feeling tired and sore a good part of the time. And because he was feeling tired and sore, he had to push himself even harder to continue the regimen—and, predictably, this further lessened his sensitivity. His pain, injuries, and limitations now got worse. After a week or so of this, he was growing discouraged, yet still determined to "get in shape" so that he didn't feel so worn out all the time. He was beginning to believe that the vitality he was seeking was lost to him forever.

Gary was now caught in the vicious circle that is too often the unfortunate by-product of using excessive force. The more effort he put into his exercise program, the more uncomfortable he became and the less vital he felt; because he felt more tired and uncomfortable, he increased his efforts, producing even more discomfort. Believing that he could break through this barrier with a little more effort, he increased his use of excessive force even more—and so it went, producing just the opposite of what he wanted.

With the help of NeuroMovement Gary learned to reduce force and notice what he was feeling as he exercised; he broke the vicious circle and a miracle happened. The aches and pains disappeared. As he felt more subtle differences in his body, he was soon exceeding his personal best both with the weights and with walking. The exercise sessions themselves became pleasurable, something he looked forward to with a great deal of enthusiasm.

EXERCISE 3   COUNTERINTUITIVE

In whatever exercise program or sport activity you participate in, choose a movement or sequence of movements in which you'd like to improve, get past a limitation, or reach your personal best. The next time you do this movement, at a time when the outcome really doesn't matter, instead of powering through it, take a moment to practice: Reduce the force by 90 percent. In some cases, it will be easier to do this first without the usual equipment—as with a tennis serve, weight training, or archery, then with the equipment. If this initially feels strange or wrong, don't worry. Keep doing the movement or sequence of movements with the least force you can possibly marshal. After a few repetitions, resume doing the same movement or sequence as you normally do. Observe whether there is change and improvement. Subtlety is the "it" that brings you to the "be here now" that your brain requires to gain the new information it needs to improve the organization of your movement for greater efficiency and effectiveness.

ENJOYING SUBTLETY IN YOUR
EMOTIONAL LIFE

Vicious circles can happen in the emotional, mental, and spiritual arenas as well as in the physical. A child's emotions are very strong, very immediate, and undifferentiated. Get ice cream: *happy*. Take ice cream away: *tragic*. There's no in-between: more refinement only comes with experience over time, with the brain growing and refining itself. Every child is like that. We are born that way. But we are also born to *divide light from darkness,* that is, to differentiate our emotions more, to go beyond "I hate you" or "I love you," or "I am happy" or "Everything is in the dumps" to greater distinctions between the extremes. To do that, we need to reduce the emotional force we are exerting and provide ourselves with opportunities to feel what is going on. As we do this, our brains create new, more refined possibilities. If we don't get enough of these opportunities as children—or don't do it later in our adult lives—our emotional lives can become stifled, or we may frequently find ourselves on an emotional roller-coaster ride.

What we know about the experience of vitality is that it includes the ability to feel a very wide range of emotions—including many subtle shades between, for example, love and hate, pleasure and pain, joy and sorrow, and so on. Adults who are limited to the expression and experience of the crude, undifferentiated emotional extremes usually find themselves frustrated, exhausted, or simply stuck. They certainly feel anything but vital. Moreover, they often get caught in the vicious circle that is the product of using excessive force: Conflicts escalate, we give up on relationships because we can't find our way through, or we struggle where we would have liked to be loving. We are like elephants in an emotional china shop. Until we are able to reduce force and allow ourselves to develop a fuller, finer, and richer range of emotions, we may very well feel that we are missing out on life, and in reality we are. After all, vitality is defined, in large part, by how much we are able to be in the present and feel the richness of our emotions. Then we can dance with life, powerfully and effectively.

Some years ago, I had a client who was an administrator at a university thirty miles from my center. Carla was an intense, wiry, and very athletic woman who had accomplished much in her thirty-two years. Even though she came to me for a knee injury she'd suffered as a result of overtraining for a tennis tournament, it ended up to be much more than that. What I first noticed about Carla was that she appeared to be in abject despair over the possibility of not being able to compete in the tournament. It seemed to me that her emotion was out of proportion to the importance of the tournament. But I did my best to reserve judgment until I learned a little more about her.

It did not take long to discover that Carla had been training with excessive force, leading to her present injury. Moreover, everything she did she seemed to do to the extreme; she talked louder and faster than was necessary to be heard and understood. Though she had a small and muscular body, she moved as if she were having to force her way through a crowd. Her movements tended to be forceful and jerky rather than smooth.

As I worked with her, using NeuroMovement principles, she began to slow down, feel more, and refine her movements. We were, in fact, breaking a vicious circle she'd been caught up in with her training for the tournament. The pain of her knee injury was quickly diminishing, and she was feeling more optimistic.

During our third or fourth session, Carla confided that other tennis players in her club hated to play with her. When I asked her why, she answered that it was because she was so intense. With a little more probing, she told me that she hated to lose, and she admitted to expressing herself freely, which to her meant shouting, stomping off the court, and even smashing her racket in a couple of cases. It was easy to imagine this, since it seemed so consistent with her overall demeanor. When I asked her if this was something that bothered her, she admitted that it did. "I embarrass and exhaust myself and I end up feeling horrible," she said. "I also wish I had more friends."

In Carla's work with me, she had become increasingly sensitive to her physical movements and was enjoying greater success by reducing the force she used when she was playing or training. Because she was having success with reducing force in the physical arena, it was easy to suggest ways that she might apply the same practices in the emotional arena. For example, I asked Carla to vividly recall a time when she lost a game and ended up being upset, yelling and stomping. She did. I saw her breathing change and her muscles tighten. I then asked her to remember a time when she was even more upset. She now recalled a time when she got so upset she broke her racket. Then I asked her if she could imagine being even more upset. This was somewhat challenging, but she did it. I pointed out that she could have a range in how upset she felt and how she expressed it. I had her imagine being upset, but less, then more, then less again. Each time, she imagined another set of reactions.

When she stood up at the end of the session, she was elated. She said this was the first time she had felt she could have emotional choices and the dignity that comes with it. Over the next few weeks, Carla became more and more subtle emotionally, and her extremes of emotion began to even out. She was feeling more relaxed in her relationships with coworkers and had made a new friend. Her success in both the physical and emotional arenas broke the vicious circle of injury, embarrassment, and frustration. She had moved into a circle of newfound vitality and had escaped what she described as being "held hostage by my own intensity."

Carla's example is perhaps unusual, but it is not so unusual to discover that as we reduce force in one area of our lives, we gain benefits in another. It is important to appreciate how these principles and practices can apply to our emotional life. As children, we need the opportunity to evolve and differentiate emotionally, but that process of development doesn't have to stop there. It should continue throughout adulthood and is integral to the amount of vitality we are able to enjoy in our lives. The more we are able to notice subtle emotional differences in ourselves and others, the more we can act in the now and do so creatively and lovingly.

Vitality is very closely linked with our emotional lives. Just as with movement, we can remind ourselves, throughout each day, to intentionally find opportunities to reduce excessive emotional force and as a result be able to notice and feel more about our emotions. In the process, your brain will come up with new distinctions and possibilities, which then will open up the opportunity for you to further reduce force and become emotionally creative.

Subtlety Feeds Intelligence

Forceful, crude, and undifferentiated mental activity can manifest itself through our ideas, beliefs, and prejudices. For example, consider statements such as: "The only way to achieve success is the way my father taught me," or "Young people are irresponsible," or "All French people are mean," or "You are either with us or against us." These broad generalizations are overly simplistic and express the speakers' biases and long-held beliefs. They are examples of stuck thinking, not the inventive and flexible work of a vital mind.

Thinking is a form of creativity. It is discovering relationships and making up something that wasn't there before. But our thinking is greatly limited, if not stopped altogether, when we use crude, undifferentiated thinking that is a form of mental excessive force. With excessive force, our brains cannot perceive fine differences, and notice or invent options. True intelligence requires us to make finer and finer mental distinctions. Only as we develop these abilities can we discover and create new, more-complex relationships that give us greater freedom, allowing us to better match the requirements of the moment. We never know what distinction will make the difference, but we know that we need distinctions to make a difference.

EXERCISE 4   BOOST YOUR INTELLIGENCE

You may have noticed a form of force that occurs in our thinking. It happens whenever we overgeneralize with words and phrases such as *always, never, every time,* and *all,* as in "All men are . . ." or "All women are. . . ." It occurs when we preface a statement with "Every time I ask you to . . ." or "You never . . ." or "This is the *right* way to . . ." or even "Here we go again! It's always the same." Next time you find yourself using any of these expressions, in your mind or with another person, stop yourself and take a moment to see whether you can refine your thinking. Question yourself: Is that really so? Think of other options, other possibilities, or instances in your past when your experience was a bit different from these generalizations. Experience how you begin to fill the space of that thought or belief with a richer, more vibrant tapestry of possibilities as you bring more life to your thinking. Have you known someone who has acted unlike your belief? Has there ever been a time when you have experienced the opposite of your belief? If not, just try to argue the other side of your belief for a few minutes.

INTUITION AND SUBTLETY—ANOTHER WAY TO A FULLER LIFE

As we gain the ability to perceive subtler differences, we expand our intelligence. Our brains are able to make use of subtler and subtler stimuli, to be inventive and create new connections, possibilities, and solutions. This ability to feel finer and finer differences is also at the heart of what we call *intuition*. Sometimes we are aware of what it is we perceive that leads us to our intuitive insights, but most times it happens subconsciously. Intuition enriches our experience of life and gives us a lot more to dance with. We are not limited to what we already know or bound to the existing patterns in our brains. At times, intuition can even be a lifesaver.

I recently heard the story of Juan Fangio, the champion race-car driver, who during the 1950 Monaco Grand Prix found himself braking as he exited a certain tunnel, instead of accelerating as he normally would. Because of this, he was able to avoid a serious crash that had occurred around the next corner, which was invisible to him at the point where he braked. At first, he was unable to explain why he had braked instead of accelerating. In a dream a few days later, he discovered a very subtle image that had signaled him to do what he did. He was a popular driver, and in the past people at the sidelines along the road always cheered when he emerged from the tunnel. On this day, however, they were looking in the other direction, farther down the track where the accident had occurred. Because his brain was able to perceive this subtle alteration in his usual experience, he subconsciously realized something was wrong and responded by braking instead of accelerating.

We generally think of this kind of "intuitive" knowledge as mysterious or somehow outside us. In my own experience, I am convinced that it occurs in those areas of our lives in which we have the greatest knowledge and subtlety. Sometimes this is in an activity that we are engaged in. Sometimes it is in the wisdom we have of our own bodies, minds, emotions, and spirits; after all, we live with them twenty-four hours a day. But the skill that gives us access to an increasingly wider range of knowledge and possibilities is subtlety—reducing excessive force so that we are able to notice and discern increasingly refined differences.

In everyday life, this ability to notice subtler and subtler differences brings us closer to life, closer to the now. And it is in this richer connection with each and every moment of our lives that we discover our greatest vitality.

EXERCISE 5 SUBTLETY

WHAT'S YOUR VITALITY QUOTIENT?

On a scale of 1 to 5, rate yourself on each of the following statements, with 5 being always, 3 being occasionally, 1 being never.

1. I often question the truth of the belief that there is no gain without strain.

2. Whenever I am exercising, I know to stop pushing or forcing myself when I experience difficulties or limitations.

3. Whenever I feel a disagreement or conflict arising with another person, I back off on my emotional intensity to better hear, feel, and see what the other person is trying to communicate.

4. When I find myself repeating and being strongly attached to the same thoughts, ideas, and beliefs, I back off and try on fresh perceptions.

5. I find comfort and joy when I reduce the intensity of my effort and be *in the now.*

6. When I feel stuck, I pause and try *less hard* as a way to access my creativity.

7. I like to lighten my touch as a way to enhance my own and my partner's sensual experience.

Score Yourself
24–35 points = high
15–23 points = medium
1–14 points = low

Go through the seven statements above and choose the ones in which you scored the lowest. Take some time to think about ways to improve your scores in those areas. The statements themselves will guide you.

Four

Variation—Enjoy Abundant Possibilities

If I were to wish for anything, I should not wish for wealth and power, but for the passionate sense of potential—for the eye which, ever young and ardent, sees the possible.

—Søren Kierkegaard

Many years ago, Dr. Feldenkrais was traveling on a train from Jerusalem to Tel Aviv. Facing him was a man reading a newspaper. But he was holding his newspaper upside down! Dr. Feldenkrais saw that the man's eyes were moving and that he was nodding his head from time to time, indicating that he was apparently reading.

"Are you reading that newspaper?" Dr. Feldenkrais asked, unable to figure out what was going on and too curious to let it go.

"Yes, of course," the man replied, surprised.

"But you're holding it the wrong way," Feldenkrais said.

The man put down the paper and with a puzzled expression asked Dr. Feldenkrais what he meant.

With the man's permission, Dr. Feldenkrais turned the paper around 180 degrees and said, "This is the right way."

"Thank you," the man said, obviously a little mystified by this exchange, as he resumed reading the paper.

Now even more curious, Dr. Feldenkrais asked the man where he had learned to read. The man put down his paper and explained that he had grown up very poor. At the school he attended, they had only one Bible for the whole class. The children learned to read sitting in a circle with the Bible placed in the middle. They learned to read from wherever they were sitting at the circle, with the Bible always remaining in the same position at the center. For the young readers sitting around the circle, there simply was no up, down, or sideways for the print on the page. There were as many variations in the children's views of the print as there were positions in the circle.

When Dr. Feldenkrais first told me this story, I immediately shared it with my father, who nodded knowingly. "This man you speak of must have come from Yemen," he said.

"How did you know that?" I asked.

"I have known this growing up," my father said. "Children who came from the small villages in Yemen were all exceptional readers, and they could read as well from one angle as from another. The position of the text made no difference to them."

What my father told me made perfect sense. To the man on the train, there was no "right way" of holding the paper. One way was pretty much like another for him. He was so comfortable with reading the paper upside down that when Dr. Feldenkrais tried to correct him, the man was genuinely puzzled.

I've always loved this story because it offers an important insight about the nature of our brains, our amazing human capacities and the fourth NeuroMovement Essential—*variation*. Brain re-search has shown that *variation*—think of it as the opposite of *repetition*—actually increases the *synapses* in the brain. As synapses increase so, too, do the number of connections between nerve cells. This expands the brain's potential for learning new things and for quickly adapting to new and challenging situations. My own experience has convinced me that this ability to increase the number of synaptic connections through variation continues throughout our lives.

EXERCISE 1   READING UPSIDE DOWN

As you read this book, experiment with variation. Turn the book upside down or sideways from time to time and read it like that for a while. See if it gets easier very quickly, and then, when you go back to your normal way of reading, take note of any unexpected changes or improvements.

The importance of variation is the subject of a very interesting research project. A group of brain researchers asked if physical activity alone could produce changes in the brain. They set up four separate groups of adult rats that would be engaged in four different kinds of activity. The first group, called the "Mandatory Exercisers," was put on a treadmill for a total of sixty minutes per day. The second group, the "Voluntary Exercisers," had an activity wheel attached to their cage that they used frequently but on a voluntary basis. The third group, the "Acrobats," had to go through a complex obstacle course. While not very physically challenging, this course had lots of variations. The fourth group, the "Cage Potatoes," had no exercise. Researchers looked at two possible changes: (1) the volume of blood vessels in the rats' brains, and (2) the number of synapses, that is, connections per neuron. The Mandatory Exercisers and the Voluntary Exercisers showed higher densities of blood vessels compared to the other two groups that had less physical activity. But it was the Acrobats that scored highest in the increased synapses per nerve cell. The conclusion: Variation is essential for the continued growth of the brain.

Variation is life giving. The brain either continues to grow or it withers and begins to die. This withering process will begin to show up as rigidity, pain, loss of flexibility, feelings of discouragement, even low levels of depression and a tendency toward an increasingly inactive life—all things that we associate with loss of vitality. The good news is that your brain welcomes variations and is at the ready to resume growing new connections no matter what your age or current condition.

When you allow yourself lots of variations, your experience will be rich, and you will be developing resilience and flexibility along the way. Just as with the man from Yemen, whose reading skills were expanded by variation, you will expand and deepen your capacity for easily adapting to further challenges that life is sure to present. I like to tell my students and clients that variations will keep them young and vital in body, mind, and spirit. New information—provided by variation—is as much a requirement for our brains as air is for our lungs. Without variations, we end up feeling limited, inept, and stuck. Sometimes the signs are subtle, such as not wanting to get down on the floor to play with our child or grandchild. Others extend to feeling bored or even mildly depressed. We become like automatons, rigid in our thinking, in our emotional capacity, and in our bodies—a state of being that we all so dread.

Even if everything in your life is "good enough," or is going along pretty well, or maybe "couldn't be better," be on the lookout for opportunities to introduce variations into whatever you are doing. Experiment with bringing variations into your everyday activities, whether you are standing at the sink washing your hands, calling a friend on the phone, making love, or learning a new sport.

BIG GAINS, NO PAIN

Jill's husband, a successful executive and passionate golfer, was spending more and more time on the course, even during their vacations. Not wanting to become a "golf widow" like many of her friends, Jill decided to take golf lessons. By her own account, she was a "clumsy and nonathletic person." Jill was having a tough time.

She'd had NeuroMovement lessons with me before for back pain issues, so she called me up and asked if I could help. When she came in, I asked her to show me how she held the golf club and how she swung it. I immediately saw how stiff she became, clinging to the club as if her life depended on it. This, she explained, was "the right way"—the way she was shown by the golf pro. I realized that she was taught with no variations.

I immediately began guiding Jill through extensive variations. Many of them would seem silly or just downright wrong for anyone who knows anything about golf. Jill trusted me and followed my suggestions. She held the club with only one hand, then the other. She reversed the normal position of her hands on the club. She swung the club one way and then the other, moving her head to one side and then to the other. I even had her lie down on the floor, holding the club toward the ceiling and carefully swinging it. I had her swing the club with her back slouched, then arched. I had her swing it and let it fly through the air.

She soon resumed her lessons with the golf pro and even dared to tell him about some of the work she'd done with me. To both her and her teacher's amazement, her game improved exponentially. Today, she is a fine golfer who can keep up with her husband on any course. What's more, she has actually learned to really like the game. What was it that turned things around for Jill? It was the variations I gave her to do. They gave her a wellspring of information necessary for her brain to develop a skillful swing. Any time we want to acquire a new skill, or improve on an existing one, such as how we speak to our children, how we cook, how we walk and balance, how we do yoga, or even how we drive our cars, our success will depend on our bringing in lots of variations—new information for the brain to work with.

One of the world's foremost minds in movement science, the late Russian researcher Nicholai A. Bernstein, stated that when we need to learn something new, or improve upon what we already know, we get there through a series of variations. It is these variations, not the effort to duplicate and repeat a *correct* pattern, again and again, that help the brain make selections, figure things out, and evolve. When setting out to learn something new or improve an old skill, it is good to remember his words, that "motor skill is not a movement formula imprinted somewhere in the brain. Motor skill is the ability to solve one or another type of motor problem. It is the ability to find a solution across a range of variations." This same principle holds true for all aspects of ourselves—emotionally, mentally, physically, and spiritually.

Why Change If It Ain't Broke?

We've all heard the saying "If it ain't broke, don't fix it." There's certainly not much room for variation there! And yet, there's a temptation to follow this aphorism, though we may try to make light of it. Over time, we begin excluding variations from more and more areas of our life. Things may be working fine—the sex is still great, our business or career is going well, our kids are healthy and happy. It's hard to argue that anything needs to be fixed. However, no matter how well we're doing, if we neglect to bring new variations into our lives, unbeknownst to us, the process of deterioration and loss of vitality will have begun.

Intentionally bringing new variations into our lives is like applying a magic salve. Immediately, new opportunities and new possibilities open up to us that we didn't even dream were possible.

In an article titled "The Plastic Human Brain Cortex," Alvaro Pascual-Leone and colleagues from Harvard Medical School discuss recent groundbreaking research exploring the plasticity of the brain—its ability to make new connections and create new solutions. They argue that this plasticity, which is an intrinsic property of the human brain, provides the ability to adapt and invent, enabling us to transcend our own restrictions and limitations.

A lot of what we know we learned during the early years of our lives—walking, talking, communicating, loving, thinking, and what it means to be in relationship. If we were lucky, most of it worked well enough for us at the time. As life goes on, the demands keep growing, changing, and becoming increasingly more complex. When we continue to try to apply the same old skills, we are bound to fail. The place we have all experienced this is in bringing childhood behavior into adult relationships. When we see our youthfulness slowly turning into limitation and rigidity, we often don't stop to realize that it is because these older abilities are no longer meeting the current requirements of our lives.

My friend Randy, who is a corporate life coach, told me the story of a successful executive she was coaching. He and his wife had recently had a baby, their first child, and their previously harmonious marriage was on the rocks. Randy told him to think of their prebaby relationship as a cup filled with water. Everything worked well for them before the baby came. The cup contained their relationship nicely.

"Now think of your newborn as a watermelon," she told the executive. "What you and your wife are trying to do is squish that watermelon into the cup. It doesn't fit, and it is messy!"

It was time to change the container to accommodate the couple's relationship and meet the incredible demands of the new family member. This change would come about by introducing a multitude of new variations into their lives—new brain resources for creating a bigger, more vital container for all three of them.

Our brains are always ready to form new patterns and solutions, if only we approach life with a willingness to welcome new variations. In the words of Michael Merzenich, M.D., "We are just beginning to realize that the adult brain is more dynamic than static. It continually shapes and reshapes itself from experiences throughout life." It is so very clear to me, from having worked with thousands of people, that it is not the progression of our years nor bad luck that causes us to lose our vitality. When we introduce lots of variation to what we do, think, and feel, we begin making changes that improve our lives and revive our thrill with life.

MOVING FORWARD WITH VARIATION

A while back, I had the opportunity to work with a well-known baseball player, a pitcher, who suffered from debilitating pain in his right shoulder. During the first NeuroMovement session, I asked him to tell me what he did to stay fit and continue to improve his skills. Aside from a lot of practice pitching, he said, he had a rigorous routine he followed in an attempt to build up his strength, stamina, and skill. I was stunned when he told me about the hundreds of repetitions he did every day, mostly "crunches," some weight lifting, and a bit of stretching. When I asked him what he was trying to achieve from such workouts, he explained that much of it had to do with developing a flat, "washboard" belly and a really hard body. He truly believed this routine would ensure his future as an athlete. I pointed out that this kind of workout could tighten up and limit the movement in his back and shoulders in such a way that he could easily injure his right shoulder. "Oh, I've already had surgery on that shoulder," he said. In fact, he told me that this was part of the reason he worked out so hard—to regain his strength and mobility.

When I observed this young man pitching, I saw that the way he was throwing would cause him pain, especially given the huge number of repetitions required to throw the ball in each game and over a whole season. Patterns that had perhaps served him very well when he first began pitching had become so limited and compulsive, because of his practice, that they no longer met the demands now being made on him.

As we spoke, he happened to mention that once a year he took a break from training to go skiing. During that time, he was free of pain and felt happier. He couldn't understand why. I told him that the way he moved his back and shoulders was good enough for his skiing, so his right shoulder ceased to hurt in that particular activity. But the way he was using his body when he pitched required more freedom of movement in his back and more refined coordination. That meant experiencing new variations and integrating new ways of moving. Hundreds of crunches a day would never provide that.

I explained that experimenting with many variations not only allows us to develop new and more effective patterns, but also to perceive subtler and subtler differences. As I guided him through a wide range of new movement variations, he quickly gained improvement in his movements and was able to distinguish differences between his old patterns and new ones. It took him a bit longer to give up the belief that he needed to do hundreds of crunches each day. But as he introduced more variation into his daily training, he gained benefits that his more-limited regimen had never produced. Not only did his pain diminish and then disappear altogether, but his game also improved.

What happened to the pitcher is what happens to us when habitual patterns dominate our lives and squeeze out the all-important aspects of variations that keep us alive and well. The good news is that you can reintroduce variations into your life and reverse the process. First, it's important to understand why we often stop providing our brains with the variation they crave.

EXERCISE 2   YOUR TOES ARE NOT THAT FAR AWAY

Many of us have tried to touch our toes while standing, just to discover—again and again—how out of reach they are for us. Let's see if introducing just a few variations will make a noticeable difference. Experience how variations can open the door to new flexibility and a sense of youthfulness any time you choose to bring it to whatever you do.

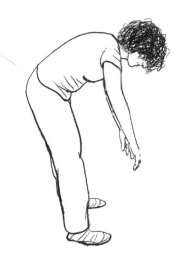

1. Stand up, spread your feet comfortably, gently bend down, and let your hands move toward your feet. Notice how far you go, without forcing, and come back to standing.

2. Stand, spread your legs comfortably, bend your knees a little, and put your right hand just above your right knee, on your thigh. Put your left hand just above your left knee. Then lean on your legs with the weight of your upper body resting on your hands. Begin to round your back, and at the same time pull your belly in and look down at your belly. Then gently arch your back, push your belly out, lift your head, and look up. Go back and forth like this four or five times.

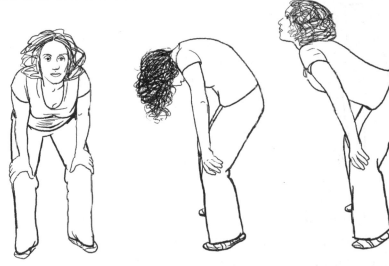

3. Come back to standing and simply bend forward and take your hands down toward your feet. Is there some change already?

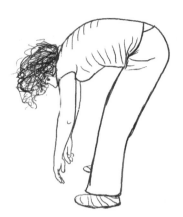

4. Stand with your feet spread, your knees bent a little, and this time lean with both hands on your left leg, just above the knee as before. Very gently and slowly round your back and look down, then arch your back, free the belly muscles—push them out—and look up. Go back and forth four or five times. Then stand and rest for a moment. Feel how you stand.

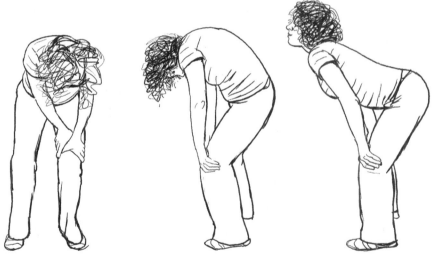

5. Stand with your knees a bit bent and spread, and this time lean with both hands on your right knee. Very gently and slowly round your back and look down, then arch your back, free your belly muscles—push the belly out—and look up. Go back and forth four or five times.

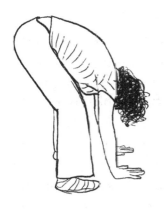

6. Stand up with your feet spread comfortably and simply bend down and feel if you can bend more easily and farther than before.

Are your toes closer to your hands? With variations provided by this exercise, your brain got the information it needed to figure out how to let go of tight muscles and tendons. You were able to quickly and safely accomplish much more than you might have accomplished by "stretching."

It's Never Too Late

When a healthy child starts doing even one simple activity, within a short period of time, the activity starts mutating, shifting, and changing. Visualize for a moment a one-year-old baby in his crib, holding on to the railing, standing up and squatting down. Each time he squats, he will do something slightly different with his knees. He'll drop them to the right or the left, or only one knee will flop down, inward or outward. Standing up, he will sometimes place his soles flat on the mattress; at other times, he will stand on the sides of his feet and occasionally even on the top of his feet. By doing these variations, the child floods his brain with new information, and possibilities to choose from that lead to his ability to stand up and walk.

As adults or as children, it is through variation that we have the opportunity to make new discoveries. We have to discover how to grab an object, how to say, "I love you," how to sing a song, how to think, and how to communicate with others. Even the simplest of these actions, like bringing a glass of water to our mouths to drink, is extremely complex. Once we know how to do these things, variation is essential for us to continue to improve, for our brains to continue to grow—and for us to be fully alive. Even the expression "I love you" needs to grow and evolve through variation. Since very little of what we can or could do is prewired, the many variations we might encounter in our lives become the essential bits of information and experience from which our brains form our unique ways of being in the world.

The adult brain is poised to respond to variation just as the child's brain is. At any age, our brains thrive on variation, with the formation of new connections and possibilities; if deprived of variation, we begin to lose neural connections. In some respects, your brain is not so much different from your thigh muscles, which will lose strength and mass, ultimately leaving it in a weakened or even atrophied state if movement becomes restricted for too long. The same is true for the brain. When fed with new information through variation, it quickly forms new neural pathways and connections.

As adults, when we give ourselves permission to play with and vary how we do things, we discover that we are as vital, energetic, and interested in life as when we were children.

No matter what the skill, be it a yoga pose, solving a math problem, playing an instrument, cooking, or communicating with a loved one, without variation you are likely to experience limitation, rigidity, hopelessness, and injury creeping in.

When we are engaged in providing opportunities for a wide range of variations, the world is full of possibilities, and our brains are working hard, sorting out all the new information, trying this and that, and discovering fresh ways for us to be and act. And that is how we can continue to be vital, starting right now.

EXERCISE 3 SMALL VARIATIONS, BIG TRANSFORMATIONS

Here are some examples that show how to introduce small yet powerful variations into your daily life. You can take these examples to inspire you in creating variations in any area of your life.

COMMUNICATION. Can you think of someone with whom you have a recurring breakdown in communication—your spouse, your child, a friend, your boss, or your employee? Next time you find yourself stuck in the same old pattern with that person, pay attention to your words, your tone of voice, and how you formulate your sentences.

Think about whether you are saying the exact same things you have said before. Is your reasoning the same as always? Are you blaming? Are you apologetic? What is your tone of voice?

When you are away from the situation, you might want to make some notes about what you observed. Then begin playing with variations. Try different ways of structuring your sentences. Change your reasoning. Experiment with different tones of voice. Then, the next time you are in the same situation, try out some of these new ways and observe the outcome. Adopt the ways that work well, and keep experimenting to continue refining your communication skills. Make NeuroMovement a part of your everyday life.

THE YOGA STUDENT. Select a pose you want to improve and begin introducing variations to that pose. You may turn your head in the opposite direction than the usual one a few times, tilt your head one way and then the other, move your eyes to look in different directions, breathe in when you normally breathe out and vice versa, round your spine and then arch it, go half as far as you normally do, and create many other variations. Then go back and do the pose the usual way and see if it has changed. Is it easier? Better?

THE PARENT. All parents have seen their child's eyes glaze over as the parent begins saying something "important." Let's see what variations in the way you speak can do to your child's listening. You can vary the timing, the location, the frequency. You can also play with the subject matter, your tone of voice, what you say, and your attitude—blaming, threatening, pleading, humorous, anxious, curious, friendly, and authoritative.

WRONG NOTE? TERRIFIC!

Unfortunately, when we encounter variations in our lives, we too often view them as mistakes. We do something awkwardly, maybe stumble as we rush up the stairs to get the phone. We play a wrong note. We misuse a word. We make a wrong turn on the way to a friend's house and get lost. On the surface, all of those can be viewed as mistakes. But what would happen if you were to treat these "mistakes" as nature's way of presenting you with variation? You might then begin to perceive differences instead of feeling bad about yourself because something is wrong; you will become curious, discover new possibilities, and become creative. There's a wonderful quote by Ralph Iron, who said, "By our errors we see deeper into life." It is often our errors, bringing sudden, unexpected change, that provide us with the variations we need to wake up our brains.

If every experience feels, looks, and seems the same, our brains will have nothing to work with, and we will have no choice but to repeat ourselves . . . and repeat ourselves . . . and repeat ourselves. Variation allows the brain to perceive differences—the raw material for it to work with. In his classic *Textbook of Medical Physiology*, Arthur C. Guyton, M.D., makes the point that the sensory receptors—the nerve cells through which we experience all sensations—"react strongly while change is taking place. The greater the change, the more impulses are transmitted—and the more they are noticed."

The history of science is filled with examples of major breakthroughs that came about through apparent mistakes that forced people to step outside what they thought they knew. There's the often-told story of Friedrich Kekulé, the nineteenth-century German scientist, who is credited with discovering the ring structure of benzene, a major breakthrough in chemistry. After days of work in his laboratory, with mistake after mistake leading him nowhere, he sat down before the fireplace, exhausted and discouraged. Suddenly, in smoldering embers of his fireplace, he saw a perfect circle of fire, like a snake with its tail in its mouth. That image broke him away from the long, repetitive line of thinking he had been following, and he had his answer. The image of the circle, or ring, was the molecular shape of the structure of benzene that he'd been seeking.

Variations such as this—a pattern in the burning coals of a fireplace—are opportunities for the brain to make a shift, awakening us to possibilities, sometimes far outside a line of logic we'd been following. Our brains are stimulated to a new level of aliveness and excitement, and this is what keeps us vibrant and young.

THE LOST CHILD—AN EXTREME CASE OF VARIATION DEPRIVATION

Jake's story—and his amazing transformation—illustrates why variation is so important. Jake was brought to me when he was just twelve months old. He was a beautiful, healthy-looking baby, but his parents said that Jake seemed unable to move on his own. He was able to sit if his mother put him in that position, but he could not move to lie on his back or belly or come back up to a sitting position by himself. He could not roll over or crawl. Unlike healthy children his age, he did not twist to look around or reach out to grab toys. He seemed to have little curiosity, energy, or enthusiasm. The only thing Jake did over and over again, especially when he got upset, was to lift his arms up in front of himself at about shoulder height and rotate his hands quickly. What perplexed me was that his body and his muscles looked quite normal.

His mother told me that soon after Jake was born he was diagnosed with "dislocatable" hip joints—hip joints that weren't fully formed. His doctor was concerned that as Jake would move his legs and pelvis, these joints might dislocate. As a solution, Jake was placed in a full body cast for the first nine months of his life. The cast prevented him from moving his back, abdomen, chest, pelvis, and legs. The cast had the side effect of denying Jake all the usual movement variations and explorations that are part of early infancy. As a result of the severe restrictions of the cast, Jake's brain had been deprived of the rich and constant flow of information that the normal movements, variations, and interactions with the world around him would have provided.

By the time the cast came off, Jake was no longer able to generate spontaneously the random and experimental movements that he would have done otherwise. Making matters worse, all those around Jake tried to help him by making him do what a child his age would normally be doing. These well-intentioned efforts denied him the opportunity of making the many mistakes, experimentations, and variations he desperately needed to catch up. Not surprisingly, he remained clueless as to how to move.

Once I established that Jake was an intelligent and healthy baby, which he most certainly was, I set about providing him with some of the variations he had missed. Gently, I began moving Jake's legs and back in many different ways. At first, I could feel that he had no idea how to do these small basic movements, even with the guidance of my hands. But within a few minutes, it was as if his brain had awakened and started working with this new information. Quickly, he became more flexible and comfortable with these new movements. His lower back was arching powerfully for the first time. Within ten minutes, he was on his hands and knees; in another ten minutes, he began crawling.

Jake's story is a metaphor for the rest of us. The habits and rigidities we develop in adulthood eventually become virtual casts, grids of limitation that restrict how we move and think and feel. If we are to live full and vital lives, we must remove these virtual casts and reawaken our brains through play and variation.

DON'T REPEAT AFTER ME

Bob, a family counselor and retired priest in his late sixties, attended a recent presentation I made to a group of psychotherapists on the subject of vitality, antiaging, and variations. He had had his right hip replaced four years earlier. He felt an improvement from the surgery, but he still walked stiffly and suffered from pain. Physical therapy and daily exercises were somewhat helpful, but he was no longer gaining any more ground and had become discouraged. It became clear to me that the routine he had been following diligently for a few years included no variation. It was a fixed set of exercises. I knew that Bob's brain was starving for new information that would allow it to replace the old habits he had created with new ones that would ease or even resolve the problems he was having with his hip. It wasn't his age or the surgery that was causing his limitations, his pain, and his suffering. It was his brain that was still using old patterns for parts of his body—his hip joint—that had changed.

I decided to lead the whole group though a NeuroMovement lesson geared toward reorganizing and improving the movements of their legs and hips. Lying down on the carpeted floor, Bob and the rest of the group were asked to do several small movement variations with their back, head, hips, and legs. The exercises were simple, easy, and safe. Within fifteen minutes, Bob excitedly announced to me that he was able to move his right leg without pain, with a free-dom and control he had not felt for many years.

The change happened so rapidly and in such an unfamiliar way that Bob had one of those "miracle effect" moments. Then it was time to get up from the floor. Bob knew, from previous experience, that getting up from the floor was going to be very difficult and painful. In anticipation of his difficulty, still lying on his side, he lifted his top leg and kicked it in the air very hard in an attempt to bring himself up to a sitting position—something he had done many times before. It failed; the forceful movement of his leg did not bring him up to sitting. He did the same thing again, and, sure enough, it failed again. I quickly intervened and stopped him from making a third failed attempt. Instead, I asked him to reduce the force of his movements and to begin experimenting with moving his head in different directions while attempting to sit up.

Within a few seconds, he discovered that by bringing his head forward and rounding his spine a bit, he could sit up effortlessly, like a child. He looked at me with an expression of sheer amazement. It still felt like magic to him, but by this time, Bob was getting a clear understanding of what it means to introduce variations into his therapy and exercise regime. Whether one chooses to call it science or magic hardly matters. The bottom line is that it gets results, and the results are lasting. We are not static beings. Rather, we are such highly dynamic beings that even a small change—variation—can bring about dramatic transformations in our lives.

PAIN IS JUST A REQUEST FOR NEWS

When we were children, variation was just part of everyday play. But way too soon we are taught to do things the "right" way. In adulthood, playing, experimenting, and making errors are seen as mistakes, being wrong, or wasting time. It doesn't take long before we have given up on play entirely in our thoughts, our emotions, and our daily activities.

By the time we have reached our thirties, forties, fifties, sixties, seventies, eighties, or older, the dangers of being trapped in a life without variation are fierce. We have gotten far too comfortable with our routines. Our emotional range has narrowed to the point of rigidity, and our minds, unchallenged by the new, have fallen into dullness. Pain in general is one of the most common ways this lack of variation shows up in our lives.

To get rid of the pain—be it physical, mental, or emotional—our brains desperately need new information to work with. With that information, they can discover and create new ways for us to move, think, and feel that are pain free. One of the most common pains we feel is back pain. If we understand that back pain is a request for a change in the way we sit, stand, move, and think about our bodies, we can then take steps to give our brains what they need—variation.

Years ago, I was teaching NeuroMovement techniques in Freiburg, Germany. A cello player from a well-known classical quartet came to me suffering from severe back pain that was threatening his ability to continue playing. Though a brilliant musician, he was afraid his career was on the line. His pain was affecting his ability to play and his emotional expression of the music, which had once been very rich and complex.

I asked him to bring his cello to the session. After he tuned it, I asked him to play for me a few musical phrases of his choice. He was a wonderful cellist, and I thoroughly enjoyed listening to his playing, but when I placed my hands on his back, I could feel enormous tightness, rigidity, and fear. Once he was done playing, I asked him to lie down on my treatment table and gently began guiding him with my hands, introducing him to new movement variations. At first, he felt like a rock. After a few moments of working with his back and pelvis, his spine, neck, and shoulders began freeing up. I was able to easily lift his right arm up above his head, with no pain to his neck and shoulders.

Despite the obvious improvement, he seemed unmoved by the changes he'd experienced. I could see that all that mattered to him at this moment was the ability to play the cello pain free *now*! There was no time to waste.

I had an idea. I would use variation directly with his cello playing.

"Take out your cello again," I told him. I asked him if he would be willing to play an easy piece, maybe something he had enjoyed playing when he was a small child. At first, he hesitated, as if he didn't understand my words. He seemed taken aback by my request, being such a virtuoso player. I repeated my request. He chose "Twinkle, Twinkle, Little Star." Needless to say, he played it easily and appeared to be a bit embarrassed to be playing this nursery song. "Please play it again for me," I asked. "But this time I have a special request. I want you to find a way to play it badly."

He stared at me in disbelief, but with a bit of encouragement, he tentatively began playing the piece in a way he considered to be wrong. The moment he began playing, I stepped in behind him and gently began moving his shoulders, his back, his head, and his pelvis in directions that were unfamiliar to him. While he seemed quite puzzled by all this, he nevertheless kept playing. When he was done, I complimented him. "You played badly very well!" We laughed, and at that moment it was as if he came to life. Then I asked him to play the song in a different wrong way. That time, he was game, and a rich emotional expression began coming through his music. His whole demeanor seemed lighter and looser.

Once he was done, I acknowledged his accomplishment and asked him to find yet a third wrong way to play the song, and then a fourth. By the fifth request for variation, it became clear to both of us that it would be difficult to find yet another bad or wrong way to play "Twinkle, Twinkle, Little Star," so we stopped.

At that point, I asked him to once again play the piece he had originally played at the beginning of the session. As he prepared to do so, I took my place behind him. I placed my hands on his back and was amazed at what I felt. His back and his movements were now fluid and easy, the quality of his playing pristine. The emotional sound and texture were thrilling. For a moment, he turned his head and looked into my face with a beaming smile. In a tone that was both relieved and delighted, he told me that the pain was gone. He felt great.

Recognizing the transformation in himself, he asked, "How can I keep this?"

"You can't keep it," I told him, "but whenever you begin to feel stuck, in pain, or unhappy with your playing, remember how you're feeling now and intentionally experiment with different ways of playing badly—with bold variation—until you feel free of pain. Give up on thinking that there is only 'one right way' of playing. Do not be afraid of making mistakes, but think of mistakes as a shortcut to your next discovery."

EXERCISE 4 USE VARIATION TO OVERCOME PAIN AND LIMITATION

The experience of pain and limitation calls for a change in the way you are moving. Introduce abundant variation to how you move that part of your body, and also introduce variation to the way you move other parts of your body in relation to the painful one. If, for example, you feel pain or limitation in your lower back when you bend down, here are some variations you could do.

Make sure to do only small, very gentle movements. Stop for a few seconds after each variation and pay attention to any changes in how you feel.

Sit comfortably at the edge of a chair with your feet spread comfortably flat on the ground, your knees apart, and do the following movements.

1. Place both your arms between your knees and let them hang down toward the floor. In this position, bend your head and back down so that your hands move closer to the floor and come back up. Do the movement three or four times. Make sure to move

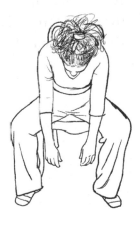

gently and slowly and see how far down you go without stretching or forcing. Sit up and stop for a moment.

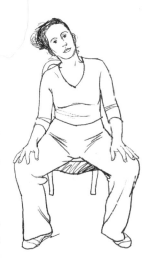

2. Gently bend your head and shoulders sideways to the right a few times. Stop and rest for a moment.

3. Bend your head and shoulders to the left a few times. Stop and rest for a moment.

4. Gently twist your head, shoulders, and back to the right, then round and straighten your back while twisted. Do the movement three to four times and rest.

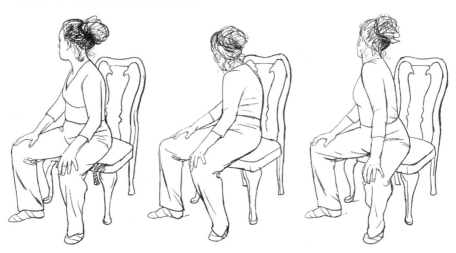

5. Twist your head, shoulders, and back to the left and round and straighten your spine. Repeat three to four times and rest.

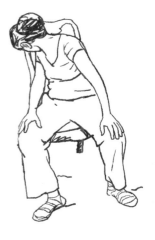

6. Round your back and pull your belly in, and in this rounded position, gently turn your head and shoulders right and left, three or four times.

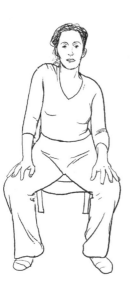

7. Sitting with your head and shoulders back in the middle, lift your right shoulder to your right ear, lower it, and lift your left shoulder to your left ear. Alternate like that a few times and stop for a moment.

8. Round your back, pulling the belly in, then arch your back, rolling your pelvis forward and pushing your belly out. Repeat a few times.

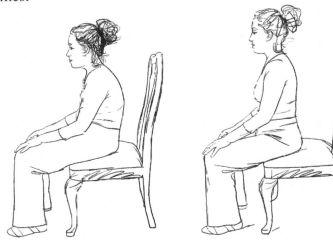

9. Now simply bend down and see whether your hands come closer to the floor without forcing or stretching, and with less pain—if you experienced pain earlier.

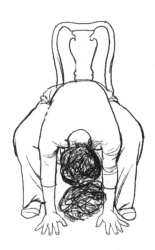

THE JOY OF MAKING MISTAKES

For most of us, the belief that mistakes are bad is deeply ingrained from early childhood. We are embarrassed when we don't do something right. We feel smaller when we mess up. In our effort to avoid embarrassment, we often learn an acceptable way of doing things, and then we stick to it. Once we have learned this acceptable pattern and feel satisfied that we are doing it "right," we keep doing the same thing over and over again. After a while, we no longer even think about it. Soon, we're like baby Jake in his full body cast. We are no longer providing our brains with the variation they need to do their job as successfully as they are capable of doing.

William Westney, a concert pianist and award-winning educator, is an advocate of variation and of making intentional mistakes. When teaching what he calls his Un-Master Class, he suggests to his students that if the music is slow, practice it fast. If it calls for evenness, make it enthusiastically uneven, with vastly varying patterns. He admits that it is challenging to give ourselves permission to go in wrong directions but when applied, it works with amazing efficiency to help people change and improve an old pattern or learn a new one.

Can you remember a time when you tried to learn a skill, failed, and gave up? It could have been an academic skill, like trying to solve a math problem, or an athletic skill, such as trying to learn to skate, dance, or play a sport. Or maybe it was an emotional skill, as when you were trying to get along with a loved one. Most likely, it wasn't that you were too lazy, not talented enough, or lacked the courage. You probably assumed—or were told—that there was a single best way to do what you were trying to do. In trying to perform that "right" way over and over again, we deny ourselves the play and exploration that would provide our brains with the variations they need in order to discover new possibilities and figure it out. As a student of mine remarked after a series of sessions with me, "All my life I have disliked my body. At fifty-two, this is the first time that I really feel I like it. I can't believe that all these new ideas and small movement exercises could make such a difference."

It takes courage to allow variations and give ourselves permission to play. Yet it is a necessity if we are to be vital and feel good about ourselves.

CREATING VARIATIONS IS NOT A HABIT

When is the last time you tried to do something in more than one way? Think about your habitual daily activities. If you are a coffee drinker, do you always scoop the coffee with the same hand? Do you press on the coffee grinder in the same way? Is the relationship of your body to the coffee machine always the same? If you are the parent of a small baby, do you always change his diapers with the same hand and in the same way? Do you always get into your car the same way? Do you always take the same route to work or to the store? Is the tone of your voice always the same when you greet your spouse or your friends? Do you discipline your child using the same words and phrases over and over again? How often do you consciously try to find new ways of doing simple daily routines? If you are like most people, the answer is *not very often.*

Creating variations cannot and never will be automatic or a habit. We need to constantly seek opportunities to vary what we do. We need to consciously choose to create variations. Otherwise old habits will always take over. Author Miguel de Unamuno said, "To fall into a habit is to begin to cease to be." If your goal is to be fully alive now, and into the future, keep reminding yourself of the magic that comes with seeking variations.

THIS STORM'S FOR YOU

Daily life presents us with ever-greater challenges, sometimes with seemingly overwhelming ones. When illness suddenly rears its ugly head, when we lose a job, or when we lose a relationship, our experience with the fourth Essential for Vitality, variation, becomes increasingly important. The more practice we have with variation, the more able we are to use it, along with experimentation, to create new possibilities and solutions for ourselves. With that ability to vary and experiment, we are often able to see stress in a new light—

not just as a challenge, but also as an opportunity to be pushed, or even catapulted, into greater realms of vitality and satisfaction.

At times, the resilience we gain through our knowledge of how to employ variation can mean the difference between having a successful life and feeling discouraged and depressed about the direction our lives are taking. Think of the cellist. Had he been resistant to variation and change, pain would have ended his career.

All around us, we see evidence of how life challenges can lead to shrinking, becoming less flexible, losing strength, memory, creativity, sensuality, and joy. If left unattended, deterioration happens to us humans just as it happens with everything else around us: Roofs leak, walls rot, weeds take over the garden, and cars cease to run. But this does not have to be. Throughout our lives, our brains constantly seek to evolve. That is the way we are designed. As humans, we have the capacity to regenerate and improve ourselves by choosing to continue to evolve.

Variation is an essential part of that process. As you continue playing with this and other NeuroMovement lessons, they will become easier to do, and you will become more and more creative. Variation does not mean relearning everything from scratch. It just means introducing small changes to what you are already doing in your daily activity and when you are learning something new. It means playing and experimenting and then playing some more. Variation will bring small and big miracles into your life.

EXERCISE 5   ENDLESS POSSIBILITIES

WHAT'S YOUR VITALITY QUOTIENT?

Rate yourself on a scale of 1 to 5, with a score of 5 meaning always, 3 occasionally, and 1 never, on each of the following statements.

1. I experiment and change the way I do everyday movements, such as getting in or out of a car, pouring milk, or holding my coffee cup.

2. I bring variations into my favorite sports or fitness activities, such as the way I run, walk, hit a ball, do a yoga pose.

3. I try different ways of speaking, including changing the tone of my voice, what I say, how I say it, and even my timing, when talking with others.

4. I bring variation into my sexual life in the way I touch, the way I communicate with my partner, what I/we do—the where and the when.

5. Before forming an opinion, I introduce variation to my thinking, and I explore different points of view.

6. I like to try new foods.

7. I like discovering new places.

Score Yourself
24–35 points = high
15–23 points = medium
1–14 points = low

You can increase your score at any time by introducing more variation into any area of your life, enhancing your vitality and improving the quality of anything you do.

Five

Slow—Luxuriate in the Richness of Feeling

Slow down and enjoy life. It's not only the scenery you miss by going too fast—you also miss the sense of where you are going and why.

—EDDIE CANTOR

Most of us are living in a world where *fast* is the byword in virtually everything we do. No matter what the product or activity, fast seems to be the added value that everyone is seeking. There's fast food, the fast track, fast turnaround, accelerated processing, instant printing, instant messaging, speed-reading, the quick fix, speedy this and speedy that, and even fast education for the youngest members of our society, babies. A radio ad I heard recently was promoting an educational program that claimed to be able to teach children to read, do math, and even solve simple algebra problems by age three. Does that mean that soon we'll see Harvard populated by seven- and eight-year-olds rushing from class to class?

We have become so focused on fast that most implications of slow have negative connotations. Indeed, when we speak of slow we automatically think of words such as *dull, dim, dumb, obtuse, boring, deadening, ho-hum, tedious, wearisome, sluggish,* or *slothful.*

In spite of our society's emphasis on fast and a tendency to be disdainful of slow, most of us know that there is also great value to be found in slowing down, in *taking time to stop and smell the roses*. Magazine ads for vacations and weekend retreats draw us in with promises of finding the perfect place to escape the busy world, to slow down, to experience ourselves in lush, sensual, satisfying ways, to think and to dream again. Yet, in our everyday lives, we still rush.

You might be thinking, "What's so wrong with fast—and anyway, what's the alternative? The way most of our lives go, there doesn't seem to be enough hours in a day to get the things done we have to do unless we rush around and do nearly everything fast." You'll get no argument from me on that point. Most of us do have very busy lives, cramming as much as we can into every twenty-four-hour period. But the vitality we are seeking can't be found by rushing around.

Rushing around from one activity to another, focusing on getting things done, we tend to place all our priorities on accomplishing tasks on our lists—doing routine housework; preparing meals and eating; commuting to work; getting things done at work; putting in time at the gym; driving our kids to soccer games, swimming lessons, and birthday parties; staying in touch with friends; taking the dog to the groomer; and so on. Are you tired yet? In the midst of it all, we become slaves to our to-do lists and become *doers* instead of *be-ers*. We give ourselves little or no time to *feel*, to more fully experience much of our lives. We forget that our capacity to feel is the very essence of our vitality. Without feeling, we become zombies or robots, and after a while we are left with a vague sense that our lives are unfulfilled, empty, lacking purpose, and devoid of anything resembling vitality.

When we're operating on the proverbial fast track, our brains will only do that which they have already done before. Going fast, we can only do what we already know. There is no room for the new. Slow is always the first step toward being more in the *now,* where we can begin to feel and experience ourselves and our lives. Slow is how we discover what it is to feel and be vital and alive, to fully participate in the dance of life. This is how we become *feelers* and *be-ers* rather than narrowing our lives to being only *doers*— and automatic *doers* at that. In our rushed lives, we are always two steps ahead of ourselves. And this is not just a perception on our part. Scientific research shows that we can either react automatically with a shorter reaction time of 0.25 seconds or less, or act consciously with a delayed reaction time of 0.5 seconds or more. If we go too fast, we simply don't have time to know what we're doing. It's as if we're not even there! We're already onto the next thing before we know it.

EXERCISE 1   TAKE A *SLOW* BREAK

Do you keep a *to-do list* in your head or perhaps written down in your day planner or personal organizer? Here's something to add to your list that will lighten your load, rather than adding to it. For each day, plan to take at least ten minutes to do something slow. Choose an activity you enjoy, one in which you can slow way down and set your own easy pace. This might be a coffee break or tea break or going for a walk. Try to be completely present during this break time, preparing your tea, fixing your coffee, walking, or whatever you have chosen to do, as if there were nothing to do but this. This time is wholly and completely your own. When you get back to your to-do list, the chances are very good that you will feel rejuvenated, more creative, and more energetic.

I WANT A LOVER WITH A SLOW HAND

Following an Anat Baniel Method NeuroMovement training, I asked one of my students how she was doing since I was aware that she occasionally suffered from hip pain. All of a sudden, Rebecca, who is in her early fifties, began giggling like a teenager.

"Anat," she said. "I don't think you have a clue what was going on in class."

She went on to tell me that once I started the class on what she called "the slow stuff"—slow movement, self-observation, and observation of others—the whole class changed. As Rebecca put it, "The whole class became sex crazed."

She went on to tell me that while she had always thought she had a great sex life with her husband, "I never thought it could be like this!"

As we talked, Rebecca became more at ease, and I asked her if she had previously understood how slow can intensify sensuality and enhance the sexual experience. She said she did know that, but she didn't really understand what it meant to be slow. She then told me how, in the NeuroMovement class, the combination of going really slow with an awareness of her thoughts and feelings was what intensified sensuality for her. Furthermore, she had compared notes with others in the class, and they reported exactly what she had experienced with the slow exercises.

"I'm lucky to have my husband taking the class with me," she said. "I'm going to make sure he continues!"

My conversation with Rebecca was an excellent reminder for me of how very important slow is in my work and in the area of awakening sensuality and vitality. I had discovered very early in my career that when I was able to slow way down the speed with which I was working with people, my clients woke up. The slower I went, the faster my clients responded. Conditions such as stiffness, pain, and emotional *stuckness* were often instantly transformed. Even when some degree of difficulty lingered after a first session, clients reported experiencing a greater vitality and a sense of new hope.

Slow gets the brain's attention, increasing its activity and forming new patterns. Slow amplifies our experiences and calls on us to *be there while we are there.* Slowing down intensifies what we feel and leads us to become more aware of our thoughts and feelings. It calls on us to experience and know what we are doing and what we are feeling. When we take the time to touch another person slowly, the slowness intensifies his or her sensations and feelings. When we touch another person in this way and give him or her our full attention, our own sensations and feelings are intensified.

When vitality fades in our sexual relationships, it's all too easy to associate our diminished sensuality with our partner. We may think, "If only he or she were more exciting!" Or perhaps there are painful moments, physically or emotionally, that need to be transformed. As often as not, however, we can reawaken our sensuality through slow. Slow is immediately available and is a simple way to awaken your brain to your sensations, intensifying them and freeing you to feel again. With slow, we don't rush past the experience of the gentle caress.

EXERCISE 2   A FEELING HAND

It is well recognized by sexologists and therapists that *slow* plays an important part in sexuality and in giving and receiving sensual pleasure. Remember, sensuality is not limited to sexuality; taking time to enjoy our sensuality is a healthy part of our everyday lives. It can be practiced nearly anywhere and at any time. This NeuroMovement "homework" is a reminder of what an important part of vitality our sensuality is.

Find an object near where you are right now. It could be a flower vase, a garment, a water bottle, or even this book. Move your dominant hand fast and fleetingly over that object. Then stop. What did you get from that experience? What are you aware of that you just felt? Probably not much.

Again, place your hand on the same object. This time, move your hand very slowly over it. Notice the texture, the shape, the temperature, how smooth or rough it is. Then stop. Do it again, slower than before. In her book *You Are Not the Target,* which is filled with exercises for awakening to our sensuality, Laura Archera Huxley says, "Simply do and feel. Let be. Be." Can you feel a qualitative difference in your sensuality as you slow down? Do you feel more? Do you connect more with the object?

Practice *slow touch* often. When you are ready, bring it into your lovemaking for enhancing mutual pleasure.

RELATIONSHIPS AND THE POWER OF SLOW

When we are with another person, slow sends an important message to him or her as well as ourselves: *You are important to me. There is nothing I would rather be doing at this moment than spending it with you.* By slowing down and paying attention in this way, we are connecting more fully with ourselves and whoever we're with—and with whatever we are doing. We are giving ourselves the opportunity to experience the richness and fullness of our lives, to discover the exquisite complexity of ourselves and the other person. I do not mean "complexity" as in a "high-maintenance" relationship; rather, I mean it in the sense of discovering the magnificent beauty and significance of our individual humanness. Great new possibilities open up to us at such moments.

One of the places we experience great challenges to our sensuality and vitality in general is in our marriages and relationships that are more than a few years old. In the beginning, there is the thrill of the new, and this newness functions like an amplifier, intensifying every thought, feeling, and emotion. Millions and millions of brain cells are *lighting up,* and it is an intensely alive time. Since newness itself is a driving force behind our experience of vitality, once familiarity sets in, we need to look for other sources to generate this kind of vitality. The good news is that newness is not the only way to do this. As our relationships move into familiarity, we have a powerful amplifier immediately available—slowness.

Familiarity is a wonderful thing in a relationship. As anthropologist Margaret Mead once said, "Having someone wonder where you are when you don't come home at night is a very old human need." But when newness fades, we are left with three options: We can look to start a new relationship; we can make no effort to reawaken excitement in the relationship; or we can deliberately deepen our experience through slow. In the latter choice, we discover the excitement of building an intimate relationship. Slow is an attention grabber that not only amplifies our experiences, but also brings us into that place of being in the now—and this is the only place we can ever truly be vital.

In his book *Flow: The Psychology of Optimal Experience*, psychologist Mihaly Csikszentmihalyi pointed out that it is "impossible for partners not to get bored unless they work to discover new challenges in each other's company, and learn appropriate skills for enriching the relationship." But how do we accomplish this?

Going slow with our lovers, particularly at our most intimate times, whether sexual or during an important conversation, not only replaces the excitement of newness, but it can also move us to wonderful new intimacies. As simple as this might seem, this use of slow in our lives fosters the creativity that keeps our relationships vital and alive. Describing the creative process, Madeleine L'Engle wrote that we are "freed from normal restrictions, and are opened to a wider world, where colors are brighter, sounds clearer, and people more wondrously complex than we normally realize." While she was referring to writing and painting, the same can be said for the creativity we activate in our daily activities when we take the time to be slow.

Caring and love take time, requiring us to slow down and let our brains catch up, to have the opportunity to feel, to be fully with the moment, to focus, grow, amplify, and create. Bring slowness to a casual caress or an evening of lovemaking. Bring it to an intimate conversation. Bring it to an evening walk on a beach, opening to the full delight of a cool breeze over your skin, the sound of your lover's voice, the shape of the clouds in the sky—an utter delight of the senses. Here, in a thousand different ways, slowing not only awakens our vitality, but also keeps relationships vibrant. It all sounds quite easy on paper, of course. However, intentionally going slow is a skill that needs to be developed. Like other new skills we've introduced into our lives, this can at first be challenging. Intentionally going slow may even require harnessing a bit of courage. Just as Rebecca did in my earlier anecdote, we need to learn to differentiate between slow and fast. Intentionally slowing down can help us perceive differences and make sense of our world when otherwise we are unable to do so. You'll remember in the "attentive-hand" exercise how you slowed down, how you were able to notice so much more about the object you touched and about your own arm and hand. This is the kind of slowing down, and increased attention and awareness, that you can create in your relationships and interactions at any time.

EXERCISE 3   SLOW LISTENING

Is there a relationship in your life you would like to improve? This might be with your child, your spouse, a friend, or a colleague. The next time you are with this person, come prepared to use what I call *slow listening* and *taking genuine interest*. To prepare, slow yourself down internally. Do this by noticing any chatter going on in your mind; slow it down and quiet it down by taking a few slow, deep breaths and shifting your attention to the other person. When you meet with this person, make him the center of your attention. Let there be nothing more important to you at this time than hearing what the other person has to say. Put on hold your own point of view and any judgments you might have, right or wrong, about what he is saying. Ask questions and, as your friend answers, take all the time in the world not just to hear his words but to notice his gestures and expressions, the music of his voice, his emotional tone, and his level of energy; take a genuine interest in him. Slow. Listen for what he is wanting to communicate with you. As you slow and listen, remember that you are not a passive spectator. Good communication is always a give-and-take. After slow listening in the way I describe here, see if you are now able to respond more to what your friend is saying, rather than with an overlay of any prior agenda you might have had. Slow gives your brain space to take in new information and create something new about the other person and what you can bring to the interaction. Make the practice of slow listening a part of your everyday life.

THE MIRACLE OF STRESS TRANSFORMED

We all have areas in our lives that cause us stress. The fear of failure is one of the most common causes of stress. We worry we won't do a good enough job or complete a task as well as we feel we should be able to, which leads to stress and tension that saps our energy. It's easy to see how this works, for example, with public speaking. Most people who are not experienced speakers immediately tense up when it's even suggested that they talk in public. The good news is that slow is a wonderful antidote to stress such as this.

When Jason's children were in grade school, he decided to become active in a parent association that was raising money to buy more computers for the classrooms. Being an engineer, he had plenty of experience with computers, but no experience speaking in public. When the parent association appointed him to give presentations at service clubs in the area, he accepted, knowing it was a great place to start their fund-raising campaign. That night, however, he couldn't sleep, and the next day he was exhausted from tossing and turning all night long worrying about what he would say at the presentations.

Over the next week or so, his wife noticed he was distracted, jumpy, and out of sorts. Finally, one evening after dinner, she asked him what was going on, and he told her how uncomfortable he was about the upcoming speech. He really didn't want to do it. She offered him some advice. As Jason told it, the first thing she said was "Slow down!" As a school counselor, giving talks was part of her job description and something she was comfortable with. She coached Jason through his fear by having him slow down, notice his sensations and feelings, and not try to escape from or deny what he was experiencing. He found that every time he even thought about the upcoming presentations he was going to do, his heart rate went up, he held his breath, and he began to sweat. He imagined that he would stand up to speak and would be so frightened that no words would come out of his mouth. Maybe he'd even pass out with the sheer terror of delivering his speech to the more than 150 people who were expected to attend his first speech. His stress levels zoomed off the charts!

Drawing from her experience with NeuroMovement, his wife had him slow *way, way down* as he allowed himself to experience the feelings and thoughts that caused him all this stress; as he did this, something quite unexpected began to occur. His fears diminished. No longer were his catastrophic ideas and feelings a mystery to him. He could now focus his attention on what he actually wanted to say. Once Jason allowed himself to experience his stressful feelings, his wife had him turn his attention to the opportunity he would have for sharing with others the passion he felt for the computer project and how it would benefit the kids. He took the time to create a mental image of what he wanted to share with his audience; he rehearsed it, slowly and carefully, a number of times. Then his stress level dropped, his heart rate went down to normal, and he began to focus on his excitement and enthusiasm for the project.

As he slowed down and became aware of these positive new feelings around his passion and commitment to the project, he felt great energy and vitality. On the day of his first presentation, he felt his fear but remembered to slow down—way down. He let himself be present with his feelings and then was able to shift his attention to why he was there. His mind cleared, and he launched into his presentation. When he actually gave the speech he had a great time doing it and he was ecstatic when a week later he got his first pledge for $500.

We often feel stress and fear because we consciously or unconsciously know that there is something in our lives that we are regularly called upon to do but are falling short of performing in a way that truly satisfies us; we need to figure out how to do it better. There are probably dozens of things we must do every day that we do okay—though not as well as we know we could. This might be anything, from organizing our desk to communicating with people, from how we stand and walk to the way we delegate responsibility at the office. We continue to do these things automatically, in a less-than-optimal way, because we have never taken the time to slow down and give ourselves the opportunity to learn how to do them really well. Sliding by and getting things done in ways we know are not quite right is a hidden but large source of low-level background stress that chips away at our vitality. One of the best signals that this is the case is when we speed up and rush through tasks.

There's a lesson to be learned from professional athletes. After a game, they often relive, in their mind's eye, portions of the game they've just played. As they do this, they can feel, and pick up on, even the tiniest deviation from what they know to be their personal best. They might not know exactly what lowered their performance at that moment, but they know that it is so. The "flaw" or "error" can be a onetime occurrence, or a habit they have that keeps happening at the same point over and over. They sense that something is missing, that something isn't quite right. Unless they slow down and take the time to alter it, that something that is missing becomes a stress point, preventing them from having access to their full energy and skill.

We all have a built-in mechanism in our brains that tells us when we are dead-on and when we are off—and everything in between. Without this capacity, we would never be able to learn and improve. It is when we don't pay attention to this inner wisdom, and instead keep speeding through life, that our vitality drains away. Well-trained athletes knows that their brains are going to keep signaling them to do something to improve—mainly, to slow down, pay attention to themselves, and follow their own inner direction to better, more-effective and empowering alternatives.

The ability to vividly feel our bodies, hearts, and minds is transformative. NeuroMovement teaches that in that space where we slow down, pay attention, and get to know what we feel, we create an opportunity for extraordinary results. The father who dreaded public speaking becomes a successful communicator, winning support for an educational cause. The athlete discovers what's missing from her performance, improves her skills, and beats her personal best. With these kinds of transformations, we not only move beyond self-imposed limitations, we also reduce background stress that drains our energy and vitality.

We all know the thrill of doing something well. As children, we get it every time we master a new skill—standing for the first time, taking our first steps alone, learning to run, learning to read, learning to skate or swim or ride a bike. What's more, our whole being yearns for that experience of accomplishment—and it doesn't end with childhood. The adult golfer seeks it in improving her game, and her whole being lights up the first time she makes a birdie. The dedicated teacher knows the feeling when his student, who has been having trouble learning to read, suddenly understands. It doesn't matter who you are or what you do; we all have to experience this level of competence in ourselves or we are soon overtaken by vitality-robbing stress.

SLOW ON THE WAY TO MASTERY

Celeste, a concert pianist, was getting ready to go on tour. Though she was well prepared, she was feeling uneasy. She was anxious, depleted, and irritable, and was beginning to feel unsure of her playing.

I had Celeste sit at the piano and play one of the pieces she was most nervous about. I noticed that in certain passages her body became quite stiff and that she held her breath. At those times, the quality of her music deteriorated. I told her to stop and start again from the beginning of the piece until she reached the first passage where she had tightened up and held her breath.

From years of experience, I have learned that when we don't know how to do something well, we tend to tighten up and rush through it, with the hope that it will somehow work out. This was true for Celeste. She was speeding through the parts that she had not yet truly mastered. She wasn't aware of what was happening to her, but she was feeling that things weren't quite right.

I asked Celeste to go back to the passage she was speeding through and to play it really, really slowly. She did, but her idea of slow was far faster than I had in mind. I asked her to take at least four times longer to play the same passage. She did this. Then I asked her to take even longer to play it . . . and still longer! At last, she was playing about as slow as it was possible to play and still have some sense of the music.

I then asked her, at the same time, to bring her attention to her body and what she was feeling. I asked her to begin moving very slowly those parts of her body where she was tightening up. At that moment, the magic happened: Celeste's playing of this passage transformed. The movement of her fingers became easy and smooth. Her growing confidence glowed in her face and her tightness disappeared.

Celeste remembered that when she was learning this piece of music, the passages she was now speeding through were the ones she had the greatest difficulty learning. By going slow, she realized she could master every single passage of the music. She no longer had to "fake it." She was thrilled. For nearly an hour, we went through all the passages in the music where she tightened up and rushed. Each time she played them, she used slow to "come home" to herself and to the music she had chosen for her concert. By the end of that session with me, she was exuberant, feeling energized and relaxed about her upcoming concert.

EXERCISE 4   THIS LEG IS NOT THAT HEAVY

We humans have a tendency to believe that the way to accomplish anything that is challenging or new is to do it as fast as possible. It's as if we think that the best way to succeed is to do whatever we are doing as if we already knew how to do it. We encounter this in fitness training, sports, exercise regimes, dance training, music training, learning a new software program, fixing something that has broken, or following a recipe in the kitchen. The thinking goes something like this: "When you are fit, skillful, and vital, you can successfully do what you are doing fast and effectively; hence, if you go fast from the start, you'll be effective and powerful." Through NeuroMovement we learn that just the opposite is true. By going fast, you deny your brain information it needs to discover how to do whatever you are doing successfully. That is why so often when we go fast, we feel like we are hitting a wall and our efforts fall short of accomplishing what we set out to do. Or we even hurt ourselves and give up, feeling anything but vital and energetic. This can happen at any age, with young children or with older, more-experienced adults. On the positive side, the remedy is simple and easy to incorporate into our everyday lives. Try the following exercise for firsthand experience.

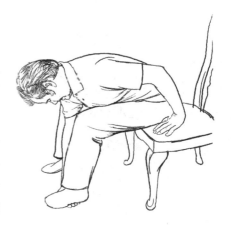

1. Sit at the edge of the chair with your feet flat on the floor and spread comfortably. (Take your shoes off for this exercise.) Make sure your knees are apart, too. Lean with your left hand slightly behind you. Bend down and slide your right hand under your left foot and get hold of the foot this way. If this is too difficult for you, get hold of your left

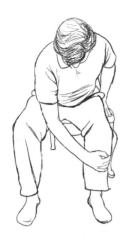

leg below your left knee wherever you can with ease. In this position, begin to lift your left foot off the floor and move your leg up. If you find it too difficult to do, don't struggle. Just stop and rest for a moment.

2. Sit the same way, then lean on your left hand on the chair behind you. This time, get hold of your left leg with your right hand just below your left knee—in front of the knee. *Very slowly* begin pulling your leg up, lifting your left foot off the floor with the help of your right hand. Just this time, take your time and shift your attention to your pelvis and to your sitting bones. Notice if your pelvis is trying to tip toward the back of the chair. The next time, before you lift your leg, begin rolling your pelvis back and a bit to the right; round your lower back while holding on to your knee with your right hand, until you feel your left leg getting lighter. At that moment, lift your leg. Put the leg back down, *very slowly,* and feel how your pelvis rolls forward. Repeat this movement four or five times. Use the time you now have, since you are moving so slowly, to *feel* how to move your pelvis and lower back so that your leg will feel lighter as you lift it. Stop, come back to neutral, and rest for a moment.

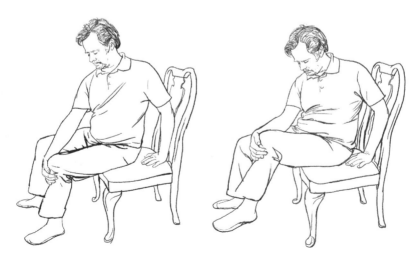

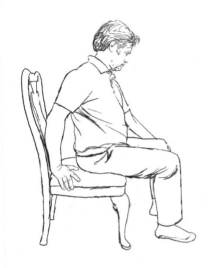

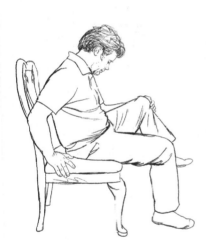

3. Sit the same way, but this time lean on your right hand behind you and with your left hand, get hold of your left leg just below and in front of the knee, and lift the left leg up with the help of the left hand this time. Move real slow, so slow that you can feel again how your pelvis can roll back, how the whole spine needs to get round, as if you are slouching, how your ribs expand in the back and your whole back moves backward and to the right in space. As you lift your left leg, let yourself exhale, and let your head bend down as you round your back. Then slowly move your left leg back down and feel how your left foot resumes contact with the floor. Do this movement four or five times. Let go of your knee and rest for a moment. Is the contact of your left buttock and sit bone with the chair different from the contact your right buttock and sit bone has with the chair?

4. Do the same movement as in step 3; just get hold of your lower leg, from in front, lower down toward the ankle, and do one or two movements, very slowly, so you have time to feel and move yourself with all the previously described details. Feel when your leg is ready

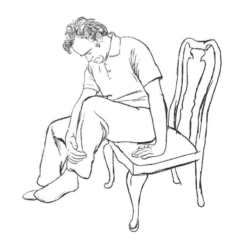

to lift easily, and only then lift it up off the floor. Only if it is easy to do, slide your left hand lower down toward your left ankle and do the movement again, holding your left leg like this two or three times. Rest for a moment.

5. Do the same movement as in step 2. Is it easier? If yes, slowly slide your right hand lower down toward your left ankle, hold your left leg from in front with your right hand, and lift the leg, slowly, so you can feel what you are doing with your pelvis, how you are shifting weight, moving your back backward and a bit to the right. Do the movement two or three times and, if easy, go a little lower with your right hand. Rest.

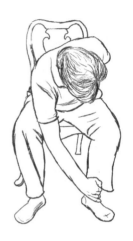

6. Again, hold your left leg with your right hand as low down as you are comfortable. Simply lift the foot off the floor with the help of your right hand, and place your foot back on the floor. Any easier than when you first tried it? Only if it has become very

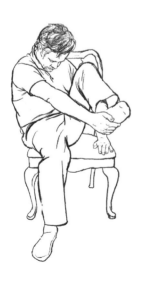

easy for you to do, place your right hand under your left foot and lift it off the floor that way. Now, try doing the movement faster. Has it become much easier? Are you lifting your left leg higher up without even trying? For a moment, get hold of your right leg with your left hand as close to your right foot as you can comfortably and lift that leg and feel the difference. Go back to holding your left lower leg with your right hand and lift the leg once again. Feel how slow, in a very short time, made you stronger and more capable.

Through slow, your brain—and you—get a chance to feel and figure out how to do well whatever you are trying to do. You become more intelligent, vital, and strong. Bring slow to your exercise or sports activity and see yourself soar. Bring slow to any area of your life in which you are learning something new, in which you want to learn how to do something better, or in which you want to bring greater ease, comfort, and vitality to something you already do in your life.

FROM SLOW TO FAST AND BACK TO SLOW

Is fast bad? No. On the contrary, when we take the time to go slow and master whatever it is we want to learn, we are able to organize our action effectively. As our skill improves, we are able to do it faster and faster. When we can do something fast, and without tension, it can be both exhilarating to do and exciting to witness. Our brains are built to turn slow into fast. Following the principles of Hebbian plasticity we discussed in previous chapters, anything we do over and over tends to become automatic, more deeply ingrained, and faster. Athletes call this "grooving." But we don't want that to happen with what we do poorly or in a mediocre way. Following this kind of groove will eat away at our vitality. Remember, there's a part of us that knows when we are not doing as well as we might—even if other people never seem to notice it.

When Celeste slowed down, she provided her brain with the opportunity to organize her piano playing in the passages that had been difficult for her. Her speed and control immediately improved, as did her vitality and confidence.

Slow is for creation and learning. Once we've mastered the activity we have set out to learn, speed can follow. There are some things, of course, that must be done with appropriate speed in order to do them well at all: racecar driving, jumping, diving, playing any stringed instrument, or simply leaping out of the way of a car that that has come racing around the corner. In music, of course, modulating slow and fast rhythms is integral to the composition.

The same is true for our daily activities. When you wash the dishes or put them away, when you fold the laundry or take a walk, slow down from time to time and you will immediately begin to feel your body more. Notice what you are doing and how you are doing it. Notice what you are thinking and feeling. This will give you an opportunity to experiment with and fine-tune what you do. After a few minutes, when you return to a faster pace, you will most likely notice that your action is easier, smoother, works better for you and oftentimes has become faster. This is a way to use a mundane activity to wake up your brain and experience greater creativity, pleasure, and vitality. It is important to distinguish between "rushing" and speed. When we skip the slow and go fast too soon, we're rushing. When we push too fast through an activity we know we haven't learned to do well, that's rushing . . . and this is frequently the cause of the loss of vitality.

To Thine Own Self Be True

One day, Judy's husband, Sam, announced that it was time to buy her a new car. They were well off financially, and he liked to trade in their cars every couple of years. Judy had been eyeing a new Mini Cooper for several months. It was small and easy to handle, making it perfect for trips around town. Besides, it was cute and stylish and even got top performance reviews in the car magazines. On the day she and Sam went to look for cars for her, he patiently stood back while she talked with the saleswoman about the Mini Cooper. He even stayed back at the dealer's waiting room while Judy went out for a test-drive. When she returned, one look at Sam put her on edge. When she asked what was wrong, he told her nothing was wrong, but suggested they should use the time to check out other cars and other dealerships.

They ended up at one of the domestic dealerships. Judy watched as Sam turned his attention to one of the cars in the showroom. He seemed very excited about it and immediately started showing her all of its features. That led Judy to believe that Sam had already decided on the car he was going to buy for her. The car was perfectly adequate, but it was not the car she wanted. By then she was feeling rushed, pressured, and tired, convinced that she knew Sam's preference. She just wanted to get the whole thing over with. With little or no discussion, she drove the new car home and parked it in the garage.

Every time she got behind the wheel, she relived that day when they bought the car. She reexperienced how she gave up on getting the car she really wanted. It exhausted her to even drive to the local shopping center. She really didn't want to be in that car. But mostly, she was upset for rushing into a decision instead of taking the time to find out what would really work for her. She had known what she'd wanted but had let her fatigue, confusion, and her desire to please her husband rush her into an inauthentic choice.

In this case, there was a happy ending to the story. She eventually sat down with her husband and they talked about what had happened. They didn't rush. They both took time to go slow and be with what they were feeling and thinking. To Judy's surprise, Sam told her that he would have been just as happy if they'd gotten the Mini Cooper. He had just gotten excited about some of the features of the other car. That led them to sharing some important personal insights that brought them closer together. And, yes, a little over a year later, Judy did get the car she wanted.

Whenever you introduce slow to your thinking, and attend to your feelings, you begin uncovering assumptions and beliefs you might otherwise never know you have. Our lives are based, to a great extent, on beliefs and assumptions. However, so often we don't know what they are. We seldom slow down enough to find out. When we do, we discover what is true for us. We are able to make choices that are authentic for us and that energize us.

Albert Einstein said, "Few are those who see with their own eyes and feel with their own hearts." Intentional slowing down is a powerful way to wake up our brains and have our feelings guide us to discover and create our own unique ways of doing things that work best for us and for those around us. It gives us the opportunity to be in harmony in our bodies, in our thoughts, and in our emotions. Being true to ourselves is what we all need to experience vitality, and NeuroMovement shows the way.

EXERCISE 5 SLOW

WHAT'S YOUR VITALITY QUOTIENT?

On a scale of 1 to 5, rate yourself on each of the following statements, with 5 being always, 3 being occasionally, 1 being never.

1. Whenever I exercise and feel some limitation or pain, I slow way down to feel what I am doing so that I can change it.

2. I often luxuriate with long, slow meals to experience the various flavors.

3. Whenever I find myself rushing, I slow myself down so that I get better outcomes.

4. When I am having difficulty with my computer, or some other object, I slow down and take the time to experiment with a variety of possible solutions.

5. When I get into a disagreement with another person, I take a deep breath, turn my attention to listening, slow my thoughts, and speak less.

6. When I touch or caress a person close to me, I slow my movements so that I can feel more and connect more with him or her.

7. As I explain something to another person, I slow down and watch and listen for his or her responses so that I can better gauge how much he or she is getting.

Score Yourself
24–35 points = high
15–23 points = medium
1–14 points = low

Go through the seven statements above and choose the ones on which you scored the lowest. Take some time to think about ways to improve your scores in those areas. The statements themselves will guide you.

Six

Enthusiasm—Turn the Small into the Great

Enthusiasm raises the artist above himself . . . in an ordinary mood one would not have been able to accomplish many of the things for which enthusiasm lends one everything, energy, fire.

—CLARA SCHUMANN, distinguished pianist, composer, and wife of composer Robert Schumann

You've probably had the experience of attending sports events, perhaps high school or college games, or a professional football or soccer match. You may remember a time when your team was behind and it looked like they might lose the competition. You felt your own energy wilting, your mood dark-ening, and you saw the players on the field reflecting the same lessening of enthusiasm. The further behind your team got, the more the players started making mistakes, missing plays they would ordinarily have accomplished with relative ease. Then the cheerleading team went to work. Their cheers and animated movements began to rejuvenate you and give you more hope and energy. Thus energized, you, in turn, rose to the occasion and began to cheer en-thusiastically, sending your renewed hope to your team, urging the players to reach within themselves to find new resources. Soon your team was playing much better. And the more the crowd cheered for it, the more its playing improved.

Enthusiasm can have a powerful impact on our moods, our behavior, and our physical performance. Moreover, we can develop the skill for generating enthusiasm at will, so that we aren't dependent on external circumstances such as cheerleaders or a winning score or an uplifting event to inspire it. The metaphor of the athletic event, with its team, audience, and cheerleaders, can be useful here. We each have the capacity to play all three of the roles we see in the sports event I describe: (1) as people acting in the world, we are like the players on the field; (2) as spectators, we have the ability to observe and monitor ourselves, giving us the capacity for self-awareness and change; and (3) as cheerleaders, we have the power to encourage the player part of us to access the best we have to offer, and to instill new energy and vitality. Like the other Nine Essentials of NeuroMovement, enthusiasm is a learned skill, one that gets better the more we put it into practice.

ENTHUSIASM IS A SKILL

In the example of the athletic event, we witness the power of enthusiasm manifest as the sports team's improved performance on the field. This demonstrates, in a very real way, that enthusiasm is not just a *feel-good* technique, but also a skill to be developed and an action we can take. Neuroscientist Richard Davidson states that "we can think of emotions, moods and states such as compassion as trainable mental skills." To provide a reality-based picture of this process and how it works in everyday life, consider the following anecdote.

Jeff had recently turned forty when he came to me with a shoulder he'd injured while working out at the gym. He was in a lot of pain, and his doctor told him he could be facing surgery for the injury. Jeff really didn't want to do that, so he was exploring other options.

I asked him to describe how he had managed to injure his shoulder so badly lifting weights. He confessed that during his last workout, he was quite angry and believed that he had not paid attention to how he was lifting. The injury happened so quickly he really wasn't sure what he did. The expression on his face suddenly changed as he explained why he'd been so angry. More than a year before, his father had died, leaving a rather large estate to be divided among his four sons. However, the two oldest sons had hired lawyers and were trying to exclude the younger sons—which included Jeff—from their share of the inheritance.

Jeff hated conflict, and the adversarial nature of this legal battle with his own brothers troubled him immensely. He just wanted the whole thing to go away and had hired an attorney who he hoped would accomplish that for him. He spoke of the situation as though he had very little say in what happened and was helpless to change it. In the meantime, he was feeling depleted of his vitality, a condition that he'd been experiencing since the day he learned of his older brothers' intentions.

After hearing his story, I asked him what he needed from me. He told me he wanted me to "fix" his shoulder so that he would not have to go through surgery. I then began working on reorganizing how he moved his injured shoulder. At the end of the session, most of the pain was gone and he had excellent range of motion. He took this as a sign that perhaps he would no longer require surgery, and when he left my office he was feeling very hopeful.

That night, the pain returned, and he called the next morning for another meeting with me. Discouraged and confused, he could not understand how he could be nearly pain free at one moment and then have the pain suddenly return. Though I helped him to recognize his disappointment and become aware of how it could be affecting his choices, he reverted to feeling that he would need surgery after all, just as his doctor had suggested. That thought depressed him, and he slipped further into believing he was helpless, without any choice.

I pointed out to him that the pain had in fact stopped for a few hours, and that was an important reality, suggesting that we should continue our work together before making any final decisions about surgery. While he acknowledged this was true, he kept coming back to what the doctor had told him, unable to focus his attention on the comfort he'd experienced, albeit briefly. I suggested to him that he look at the possibility that his belief that he would require surgery might be a product of his disappointment about the pain returning. He nodded, allowing that this might be true; but he argued that whether it was true or not, he didn't know what to do about it.

I then suggested the following to him: He would not only come to lessons with me, but he would also begin to see himself as an active participant. He would realize that if he were to have a healthy shoulder, he would become proactive, be open to new experiences and possibilities, and eventually learn to stop reinjuring himself. I told Jeff that in order for his shoulder to have a chance of healing without surgery, he had to acquire the skill of enthusiasm.

At first, he expressed some resistance, but then, as he considered the possibility of surgery, he started asking what he should do. I gave him gentle movement exercises to do at home. And I told him that he should celebrate even the smallest improvements, to make even the most minuscule experience of progress a big deal. While this might seem weird to him, I wanted him to know that it made a big difference to his brain, where the core of his healing would be occurring. His enthusiasm for even these tiny improvements would mark them as important, bring them to the foreground of his consciousness, and amplify them so that his brain would adopt them and build on these changes that were occurring.

By the end of that session, Jeff had made his decision. He would work with me over the next month or two and see how it went. His doctor supported his decision, and we went forward with his NeuroMovesment lessons.

There were times when Jeff still felt discouraged and he would regress, fall into old habits and experience some discomfort or limitation in his shoulder again. I told him that this was normal, something he should expect, and that he would have to learn not to dwell on the disappointment. He learned to remind himself that feelings of discouragement were normal and to allow himself to go boldly forward with his healing process even in the face of his doubts.

Acting as a coach in this healing process, I constantly reminded Jeff to stay connected with the here and now by being aware of even the tiniest changes and improvements. I kept reminding him again and again of how every time he noted a change he liked and amplified it internally—made it important—it alerted his brain to pay attention to that change so that it could do its job of creating new connections, fostering new possibilities for the healing process.

Jeff's shoulder continued to improve, and his doctor finally gave him a clean bill of health. Meanwhile, he had begun applying the same process for healing his shoulder to other issues in his everyday life—mainly, the situation with his older brothers. He became fully engaged in the legal battle, working closely with his attorney. He recognized that the pain he had felt about his older brothers' actions stemmed from his unfulfilled expectation that brothers should be loyal to one another and from his belief that he was at their mercy. He also realized that this put him in an untenable position, making him their victim and draining his vitality. He accepted that he had to let go of the belief that they or his attorney should "fix" everything and make his life okay.

He clarified what was important to him—to get his rightful share of the inheritance. He played a much more active role, strategizing, researching, thinking, and making decisions. He began upgrading not only his own energy and effectiveness, but also the energy and effectiveness of his attorney. The tide turned in his favor as he utilized the principles he'd learned to employ in healing his shoulder. He stayed the course, and acted boldly even in the face of doubts, discouragement, and fears. He learned to be more creative, allowing room for possibilities—good and bad— that he couldn't have planned or controlled.

And yes, he won his case in court. He shared with me years

later that the course of his life changed when he changed, learning to employ the principles and practices that I call enthusiasm. I occasionally run into Jeff now in social situations and am always amazed at how different he is from the time he first appeared in my office. He has taken on numerous new challenges in his business and personal life. Even though it is quite a few years later, he has an air of ease and strength, full of energy and vitality.

EXERCISE 1   SO LITTLE, YET SO MUCH—COMING TO LIFE THROUGH ENTHUSIASM

Do you know people who seem to have a knack for making the impossible possible, and for whom miracles always seem to be happening? If you were to study them closely, you would find, without exception, that they are great enthusiasm generators. They create and amplify enthusiasm that energizes whatever they want to happen. Once they get this energy going, miracles begin to occur.

Try this short movement lesson. Give yourself permission to become very enthusiastic about the smallest of changes you feel; experience how seemingly tiny changes become much bigger, more important, and with unexpectedly positive outcomes.

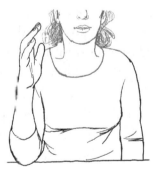

1. Sit at the edge of a chair and lean the elbow of your dominant arm on a table or desk in front of you. Bend your elbow so that your forearm is up in the air with your hand and fingers pointing to the ceiling. You are holding your wrist and fingers straight and with the least amount of tension.

2. Slowly begin bending your wrist, letting your hand and fingers go forward and down. Do this extremely slowly and gently. Imagine that your whole arm with its hand and fingers is immersed in

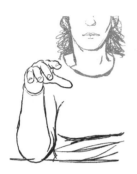

thick honey or molasses so that your hand goes forward with the palm down, real slow, and your wrist bends; then bring the hand back up—do not bend the hand backward—with the fingers pointing in the direction of the ceiling. Your elbow stays bent and your forearm stays vertical the whole time. The movement is in the wrist and hand only. Repeat this movement seven or eight times.

3. Bend your wrist and let your dominant hand go down and stay down in that position. Very slowly and gently begin moving the index finger of this hand, down toward your palm and up, away from your palm, three to five times. As you move your index finger, can you feel some movement in the palm of your hand and perhaps your forearm? Make sure that you breathe freely throughout these movements. Stop moving your index finger.

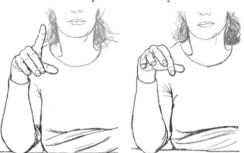

4. Still leaning on your elbow with your forearm vertical and your hand bent down, very gently and slowly (remember the honey) lift and lower your middle finger three or four times. Then do the same with your ring finger three or four times. Feel how, as you move your ring finger up and down, your other fingers tend to go along with it. Simply note this. Then do the same with your little finger three or four times. Finally, move your thumb out, away from your palm, and then toward your palm three or four times.

5. Resume lifting your hand, straightening your wrist and lifting your fingers to point toward the ceiling, and then lowering your hand down. Does your wrist bend a bit easier? Does it bend a bit farther? Are your fingers a little less tight, not so close to one another as at the beginning of this exercise? Bring down your hand and forearm and rest for a moment.

6. Remember to get interested and *enthusiastic* about the changes you feel, even if they seem small to you. In your brain, they are very big changes. Help to intensify these perceptions of differences, which help your brain discover and create new possibilities for you.

7. Again, lean on the elbow of your dominant arm, with your forearm up and vertical, and let your hand sink down, bending your wrist and staying there as before. Gently touch your thumb and little finger to form a circle. As you hold them like this, gently and slowly rotate your forearm so that your hand is moving toward your face and then away two or three times. Then touch your thumb and ring finger, again forming a circle, with your hand down all the time, and again rotate your forearm two or three times. Move your thumb to form a circle with your middle finger and repeat the movement of rotating your forearm so that your hand turns toward your face and away from your face. Do this two or three times. Finally, create the circle with your thumb and index finger and rotate your arm two or three times. Stop.

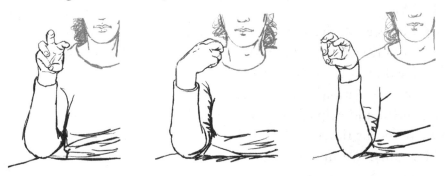

8. Again, lift and sink down your dominant hand while still leaning on the elbow with the forearm in the air. Does the wrist bend better and more easily? Does the hand sink lower? Is your breathing deeper? Are you enthusiastic about these changes yet? Are you able to make them important to you?

9. Bring both arms down to your sides. Does your dominant hand and arm feel different from the other? Perhaps longer, or lighter? Does your dominant hand feel larger and fuller? Lift your dominant arm up and feel how you do this movement; put it down, and then lift the other arm in the same way. Can you clearly feel the difference between your arms? Does one shoulder feel lower or wider than the other, with less tension? Take a book (this one is fine) and follow its contours with your dominant hand. Notice the sensations in your hand. Now do the same with the nondominant hand. Does it feel different? Is your nondominant hand clunkier, rougher, perhaps less "intelligent" and sensual than the dominant one? Which hand do you like better; with which hand would you rather type, cook, draw, and love? Are you ready to get enthusiastic about these seemingly small changes and know that you are bringing yourself more into life in this way?

THE WAY LIFE IS

Certainly, it's true that things happen in life that we don't expect, didn't plan for, and aren't the way we would have wanted them to be. We get through the tough times by employing whatever skills and devices we have at our disposal at that moment. But all too often, our vitality is diminished by it. Maybe it's just a little bit at a time, but just as dripping water can corrode steel and erode rock, the accumulation of the experiences of disappointment, discouragement, and helplessness takes its toll on our vitality. By the time we're in our thirties or forties, we may already be feeling the loss of vitality. We may experience it as a vague or even very strong feeling that "I am not where I thought I would be at this age," or "My life is slipping away and I am nowhere near fulfilling my expectations." Perhaps we even slip into a state of resignation, and that resignation itself saps our vitality even further.

The action plan that Jeff employed is the antidote to this condition. The following eight action steps—the essence of what I call enthusiasm—constitute the course of action he followed and which you can apply in every aspect of your life:

ENTHUSIASM ACTION STEPS

1. **PAY ATTENTION.** Pay attention if you are feeling disappointed, discouraged, frustrated, or in pain, or if you simply experience a loss of energy or vitality. Be aware of these feelings and any others associated with them. Notice yourself when you are blaming, venting, complaining, or feeling helpless or victimized.

2. **DEFINE AND NAME.** Identify what you are feeling and give it a name. Recognize what your unfulfilled expectations are and know that these feelings are normal and to be expected.

3. **SEIZE THE OPPORTUNITY.** Realize that your disappointment is a reflection of your vitality and life force and represents an opportunity. The gap between where you presently are and where you want to be is telling you that there is a life force in you that wants to come out and express itself. It is pointing you toward a fuller, more vital life.

4. **BE COMMITTED.** Find out what it is that you want and choose to care for it. Bring it to the foreground and choose to make it important. Commit yourself to what you have chosen and stick with it for at least a while.

5. **GET INTO ACTION.** Look around and discover at least one action you can take that will match your commitment. It can be a large or small action. Keep taking more actions and correct your course as necessary.

6. **STAY FOCUSED.** You will have moments of regression when you drift from your course or encounter obstacles. You may

occasionally feel anxiety or uncertainty. Stay focused on what you chose to care about, independent of your moods.

7. AMPLIFY. Make sure to recognize and appreciate small changes, not just what you consider big or important ones. Be willing to be bold and express your delight with small gains, knowing that this is the way large changes come about.

8. ALLOW FOR THE MIRACULOUS. Allow for the unknown and seemingly impossible to happen. The most common thing people tell me when the transformation occurs is "I can't believe it. I never would have dreamed it possible."

FROM EXCITEMENT TO ENTHUSIASM

You may remember that in previous chapters we discussed the brain's ability to create new connections and patterns. We also saw how presenting new information to the brain and calling attention to it was a key factor in waking up the brain to initiate that process. The information presented to the brain can be new or old; what sparks the process of producing new patterns is that the brain is alerted that "something important is going on." Something says, "Notice this!" A thought, action, or feeling is pulled into the foreground, distinguishing it from general background noise and making it important. I was recently reminded of this when I walked past a playground and saw a little girl hanging upside down on the climbing structure and calling out to her mother, "Look, Mommy! Look at me, look at me. Look what I'm doing."

The girl was very excited about hanging upside down and wanted her mother to see what she was doing. This is a scene that is probably repeated a million times a day on playgrounds around the world. Most children learn to hang upside down, and maybe this girl had even done it before. What is important to note, however, is her excitement, which tells her brain to "get" whatever she is doing.

This spontaneous excitement essentially gets her brain to pay attention and select the relevant connections that are being formed and to make sure to strengthen those connections. The child's performance of the action, combined with her delight, wakes up the brain, alerting it that the connections it has formed are successful.

The child's spontaneous excitement is healthy and critically important to its development. For the child, that excitement is spontaneous, often coming out of the genuine thrill of experiencing something he has never experienced before. But there is a difference between the child's excitement and the kind of adult enthusiasm we are discussing here. The young child's excitement is reactive. Imagine a four-year-old child's face lighting up when he gets the ice cream he wanted. Perhaps the child can barely contain himself, squealing with delight, jumping up and down, clapping his hands. This is also a clear picture of vitality; more than that, it is all part of the child's development, with tremendous growth and change happening within.

We can think of enthusiasm as the adult version of that kind of excitement. Enthusiasm does for the adult brain what excitement does for the child's brain. While the child's excitement is triggered by the new, and mostly from events outside of her, adult enthusiasm is initiated from within and is a set of intentionally applied skills. Of course, there is nothing wrong with excitement. It is wonderful in adulthood to be pleasantly excited by an unexpected event or perhaps by sharing our own delight with another person. But it's important to make a distinction in our own minds between excitement as spontaneous and reactive and enthusiasm as intentional and a skill. In adulthood, vitality depends to a great extent on our capacity for enthusiasm, that is, for the ability to amplify and perceive the events and experiences of our lives as important, as vital.

In adulthood, enthusiasm is a choice. It is the decision to say yes to life. This doesn't mean suddenly being a little child again and becoming indiscriminately excited about everything. In adulthood, being chronically excited can prevent us from experiencing vitality rather than enjoying its true benefits. You don't want to have the brain that you had as a child. One of the great assets of adulthood is that our brains have formed millions of connections and patterns that allow us to refine and differentiate, making it possible for us to have effective and accurate skills. This means having satisfying careers, relationships, and even leisure activities that would otherwise be impossible.

What often happens to us, however, is that we learn to develop effective and accurate patterns for our adult lives, but we seldom deviate from those patterns. The result is that nearly every moment of our lives looks like every other moment of our lives. Vitality is squeezed out, since it can't thrive in an environment of sameness. To bring vitality into our lives, our brains need to be at the ready—to amplify, intensify, and create new patterns while strengthening the ones that already work for us. And that's where enthusiasm comes in.

EXERCISE 2 BUFFING UP YOUR ENTHUSIASM MUSCLE

Think of enthusiasm as something that you *generate*. Imagine that it's a muscle you can develop and activate, rather than its being something that is only awakened by external circumstances. Like any other ability or potential, it requires learning and intentional development. Having developed it as a voluntary action, you will be amazed at how you can vitalize and bring energy to anything you are involved in.

In the next hour, choose three things to be enthusiastic about. Start with small things, such as a meal you are about to share with another person, or a new idea you are discovering as you read this book, or being in the fresh air as you take a walk. Feel how bringing your enthusiasm to these events amplifies your experience of them, vitalizing you and increasing the pleasure you get from them.

As you become more skilled at being an enthusiasm generator

with small things, choose a larger area of your life that you want to change, energize, and vitalize. For example, maybe you have been struggling with your child about homework or doing chores. Or maybe you want to improve sexual relations with your partner. Or maybe you want to make more money. To initiate the change, break down the situation into smaller parts. Begin generating enthusiasm around these elements of whatever you want to change. Do this for a minute or two throughout the day, both when you are in the actual situation or when you are just thinking about it. Observe how, as you continue to generate enthusiasm to your area of choice, and regardless of the moment-to-moment ups and downs, you and the world around you begin to transform the situation you have chosen in miraculous ways.

RECLAIMING THE POWER OF ENTHUSIASM

I had an experience with a client very early in my career that opened my eyes to the power of enthusiasm and persuaded me to explore its potentials for positive change and renewed vitality in people's lives. Lenore, a woman in her sixties, had been referred to me by another practitioner. As she entered my treatment room for the first time, she walked stiffly, as if she were in constant, unremitting pain, her body rigid, inflexible, and nearly lifeless. During an initial interview with her, I learned that she was a Holocaust survivor. Not surprisingly, she still carried in her mind and body grievous memories of her years in a Nazi concentration camp. When I asked about her present complaints, she described extensive aches and pains, and how unrelenting fear and anxiety discouraged her from venturing out of her home and participating in life. Nothing she had tried had been effective in easing her pain and her fears.

As I listened to her story, I began to join her in her discouragement and fear. Though she had come to me with the hope of making her life better, she understandably seemed to be stuck in the belief that it was simply not possible. I remember feeling discouraged. It was when I touched her shoulder to try to move her and felt how stiff and disorganized her whole body was that I thought, "Oh my God, I don't think I can help this woman!" As this thought went through my mind, I felt myself internally stopped. At that very moment, I noticed that Lenore held her breath for a long time and then began breathing very shallowly. I asked myself, was she holding her breath in response to my thought and feeling that I could not do anything for her?

I intentionally set about to change my own thoughts and feelings to more enthusiastic and hopeful ones. At that moment, it occurred to me that it was Lenore's intelligence and will to live that enabled her to survive the unthinkable conditions in the concentration camp many years before. I realized that I could help her tap into that same intelligence and life force to help her form new patterns in her brain and new possibilities for her life. In that moment, as I changed my thoughts and brought enthusiasm into my work with her, Lenore took a deep breath and began breathing freely. Just to be sure, I intentionally went back to think my discouraged thoughts. Sure enough, Lenore held her breath again. That was the last time that I allowed myself to lose my enthusiasm with Lenore. As I accessed enthusiasm for her ability to change, Lenore began to open up and respond.

As we continued working together, we emphasized small changes that were occurring, enthusiastically bringing them to the foreground. Lenore was changing very quickly. She became more flexible and fluid in her movements. Her pain eased and her outlook on life was transformed, reflecting a much more positive approach to each new moment. In my mind, it was as if she had been transformed from being a frozen statue to being a living, breathing, vibrant human being.

This was a turning point in my own life as well as Lenore's. While she turned a corner and became more comfortable, I was alerted to how profoundly important enthusiasm is in all our lives. I realized that enthusiasm is transformational for our bodies, minds, and spirits, leading to real physiological changes. With enthusiasm, movement becomes easier; we are more welcoming of the new; changes in habits happen more readily; thinking becomes clearer and more creative. In my everyday life, it was like rediscovering the joy of childhood excitement, with the addition of adult awareness and deliberately employed skills.

WHEN LACKING ENTHUSIASM

While Lenore suffered extreme hardships, none of us is immune to life's many challenges. Being human means experiencing "good" days and "bad" days, successes and failures. It also means having aspirations, looking to make our lives and the lives of those we love better and more comfortable, and using our creative abilities to express ourselves.

In adulthood, our health and vitality, as well as our ability to achieve and succeed, are very much dependent on our ability to generate enthusiasm. We lose enthusiasm and vitality for many reasons: We fail a test, a parent doesn't come through with a promise, we are passed over for a promotion, we suffer an illness, we carry a limiting belief about ourselves, we lose money in the stock market . . . life happens.

In the face of such disappointments and challenges, the lack of enthusiasm compromises our ability to make use of both internal and external resources. At the time when we most need to invent, discover, and regenerate—thus upgrading our energy—we instead downgrade our energy and lose vitality. Lack of enthusiasm at such times increases our inclination to buy into our disappointment and entrench its reality.

We are also challenged by our brain's built-in tendency to repeat existing patterns that make it very easy for us to get stuck in our routines. It is important to acknowledge the positive role these patterns play in our lives, but it is equally important to recognize that life itself is unpredictable, and each moment is different from the one before.

We need a brain that can invent the new as it relies on the old. When we are without enthusiasm, we miss out on a powerful tool that catapults our brain past its deeply grooved automatic patterns of movement, thought, and emotion. Everything begins to look and feel the same; it becomes increasingly difficult to even recognize what is new in each moment. It is very difficult to entertain ideas that are outside the most familiar patterns of our past experience. We get stuck, life gets duller and duller—and so do we.

Lack of enthusiasm can be learned and can become a habit. Enthusiasm is such a necessary part of human life that when we lose it, or we simply lack the skills to generate it, we not only drain ourselves, but also become a drain on others. The vitality and magic of life vanishes. We may then find ourselves lacking enthusiasm not only in time of trauma, great loss, or unfulfilled expectations, but also as our regular way of being.

You may remember Eeyore, the "old grey donkey" character in *Winnie-the-Pooh* whose dispirited outlook on life is unrelenting. He epitomizes what we're like when we lack enthusiasm. When Winnie-the-Pooh found Eeyore's lost tail, Eeyore said, "Thank you Pooh, you're a real friend, *not like some.*" When he saw his own reflection in a stream, Eeyore thought, "Pathetic . . . but nobody cares, pathetic, that's what it is." When Pooh Bear greeted him with "Good morning," Eeyore responded gloomily, "Good morning, if it is a good morning, which I doubt."

"Why, what's the matter?"

"Nothing, Pooh Bear. Nothing. We can't all, and some of us don't. That's all there is to it."

"Can't all *what*?" said Pooh, rubbing his nose.

"Gaiety. Song-and-dance. Here we go round the mulberry bush."

There are times in all our lives when we find a certain comfort in withdrawing from the world, feeling sorry for ourselves, and adopting an Eeyore-like approach to life. Like Eeyore, we slouch both physically and emotionally. We hunch down, drag our feet;

the tone and tenor of our voice drops and slows, and our moods become as slouchy and *draggy* as our posture. We become what a young friend of mine calls a "drippy drain." When we are caught in the Eeyore syndrome, we are opting out of new possibilities and vitality. At such times, it can take an extra effort to remind ourselves that we have a choice: We can either be enthusiastic—or increasingly *Eeyoric*. Our brains will go either way.

Science has revealed a biochemical component for depression and for a lot of our moods. That might lead us to believe that we are at the mercy of our biochemistry. However, our behaviors and action choices can also influence our biochemistry. In her book *Train Your Mind, Change Your Brain*, author Sharon Begley quotes researcher Jeffrey Schwartz, whose research at UCLA "offered strong evidence that willful, mindful effort can alter brain function," and can alter the actual chemistry of the brain.

WHEN REASON ISN'T REASONABLE

One of the subtler ways Eeyorism shows up in our lives is through the insistence on being "reasonable," using allegations such as the lack of evidence or lack of "common sense" to put a damper on any expression of strong emotions. When used in this way to discount new possibilities, reason pushes aside the yet-to-be-discovered. In this way, the cry for reason and common sense can deaden the gifts of inspiration and creativity. Einstein called common sense "the collection of prejudices acquired by age eighteen." Those early prejudices need to be transformed through inspiration and this is where the NeuroMovement lessons are invaluable.

For example, when we're in pain, we tend to focus on the region of that pain rather than on the total dynamics that may be causing it. That is the commonsense thing to do. However, by focusing on the pain, we actually amplify and intensify the neural and behavioral patterns that cause the pain and that we are trying to get rid of and replace with better working patterns.

Most of us have experienced some form of this when we have back pain. The most common thing we do is treat the back. Many have turned to surgery for such treatment, yet increasing numbers of orthopedic surgeons are giving up on performing back surgeries because they frequently don't work. Many now are referring patients to practitioners that address other aspects of the person's body and lifestyle, often with surprisingly good outcomes.

In my own practice, I often have to address enthusiasm issues rippling through a whole family. For example, if I'm working with a child, I also need to monitor the enthusiasm levels of that child's parents. If they focus on what their child is yet unable to do instead of focusing on gains she is making, they can limit or inhibit the child's further progress.

I am reminded here of a mother whose child I was working with. Little Maggie, her daughter, was six years old and was having great difficulty learning to read due to her neurological challenges. Over a two-month period, she had made great progress, but because Maggie was not yet reading at what her mother, a teacher, called an "age-appropriate level," her mother could not find any reason to experience within herself or express enthusiasm for Maggie's progress. She insisted that it was unreasonable to be enthusiastic until Maggie's reading reached the appropriate level. Unbeknownst to the mother, she was making it harder for Maggie to feel delighted and thus amplify her seemingly small, but important achievements.

Had Maggie been dependent only on her mother's enthusiasm for support and empowerment, any further advancement would have been impossible for her. As it was, however, Maggie's father began developing leadership skills for generating his own enthusiasm, and together he and I openly expressed our enthusiasm with Maggie's smallest changes. In the weeks to come, Maggie's reading abilities continued to improve rapidly. Eventually, Maggie's mother "got it" and began experiencing enthusiasm even when things were not yet "perfect."

Interestingly, the father's skills for generating enthusiasm grew with his daughter's growth and change. When he and his wife first faced the truth of their daughter's neurological limitations, both of them had become quite distressed. He told me that what he perceived as the "burden" of his daughter's challenges had "aged me twenty years." He was feeling like an old man. As he learned to further enhance his enthusiasm skills to help his daughter in her lessons with me, he had reclaimed his enthusiasm for his life and his own vitality.

Too often, behavior like that of Maggie's mother has the effect of dampening a person's enthusiasm and the enthusiasm of everyone around him or her, greatly inhibiting positive change and diminishing vitality. It's like putting a glass over a burning candle; eventually, the flame will be suffocated and thus will be extinguished. Dare to be like Maggie's father, ridiculously enthusiastic about your own life—even for the "small" and "unimportant"—and you will both foster new patterns and possibilities and feed the flame of vitality.

Intentional enthusiasm like this can be seen ultimately as an evolutionary process that facilitates greater awareness and creativity, providing us with the power to expand our choices about responses hardwired into our system. As a result, we can enjoy high levels of vitality unavailable to previous generations.

EXERCISE 3   LEADERSHIP, THE PATH TO VITALITY

Intentional enthusiasm is the heart of good leadership. Being a leader—a powerful, generative, and positive force in your own life and in the lives of those around you—is an enormous source of vitality. At work, at home, while engaged in a political debate or in an argument with your spouse or child, or perhaps upon hearing bad news, avoid the temptation to join in complaints, gossip, discouragement, anger, judgment, or despair. At the same time, understand that you are not in denial. Instead, in an authentic way, focus your attention on something in the situation to be enthusiastic about. You might even become enthusiastic about the opportunity for a better future opening up. Experience how, as you generate enthusiasm and upgrade your own energy, the vitality and enthusiasm levels of everyone else around you go up.

ENTHUSIASM AND FREE CHOICE

Many habits that reduce vitality originate with survival mechanisms that we are born with, such as the automatic tendency to be alert to danger. Crossing a street, we are watchful for dangers, such as a car turning a corner or a car driving at a high rate of speed. No one would argue the importance of being alert to what poses a potential danger to our physical well-being. But that same automatic reaction has slipped into our social, intellectual, and emotional lives, quite beyond sheer survival responses. We now find it in our tendency to focus on what's wrong in ourselves and others, and in finding fault or danger wherever we look. It shows up in behaviors such as gossiping, being hypercritical, and in blaming instead of seeking solutions and generating new possibilities. All of this can add up to depression and a dark outlook on life, to say the least, thus reducing our energy, stopping our creativity, intensifying our anger, and draining our vitality. The good news is that we also possess the capacity for recognizing what is happening to us through observing our own behavior, feelings, and emotions and change them through purposeful enthusiasm. In that respect, purposeful enthusiasm is at the cutting edge of our evolution, away from more automatic responses to our experiences. In a very real way, purposeful enthusiasm changes the hardwiring of our brains and creates new possibilities that otherwise would not exist. As Michael Merzenich says so beautifully, "Moment by moment we choose and sculpt how our ever changing minds will work, we choose who we will be in the next moment in a very real sense, and these choices are left embossed in physical form on our material selves." Even as we retain our inborn survival responses, with the capacity to recognize and respond to dangers and act in an automatic fashion, our brains are evolving and we are upgrading the use of our brains; we gain the freedom to create choices and be more discerning and effective.

The evolution of greater skills to upgrade our brains does not take place in a vacuum, nor does it happen automatically. All things in the universe move toward states of greater *entropy*, that is, toward greater disorder and less definition. However, energy can be invested to move us toward greater organization; this is known as *negative entropy*. One prime example of *entropy* is that Earth's energy is constantly being depleted; at the same time, it receives energy from the Sun daily, which plants and all living things on Earth use to grow and thrive—which is *negative entropy*. Another example is the way a flower dies and soon disintegrates (entropy) but simultaneously deposits seeds in the soil that contain highly organized energy (negative entropy) that can grow new plants. Our universe is constantly shifting through cycles of entropy and negative entropy—and so do we.

When we exercise our ability to generate enthusiasm, we are consciously and deliberately upgrading our brain's capacity for greater definition and order. Our brains will do what we train them to do. When we introduce the skills we're exploring here, we train our brains to increase order in the face of the natural pull toward deterioration and loss of vitality. Once we have these skills, we can choose to upgrade the quality with which we do any of our daily activities. We learn, for example, that we use roughly the same amount of energy when we speak in an encouraging way to another person—spouse, child, friend, or coworker—as when we speak to them in a critical and discounting way. The long-term effects of those exchanges—and the drain on our vitality—will be worlds apart. We actually expend more energy when we are upset and discouraged while trying to fix a problem than when we are calm, intentional, and enthusiastic about the opportunity. The difference is in the quality of organization that our brains generate as we attempt to solve the problem. In most cases, a professional tennis player will exert less energy to hit a superior serve than when she hits a sloppy one. The reason is in the refined level of organization that her brain has attained.

EXERCISE 4   ENTHUSIASM, GENEROSITY, SPIRITUALITY

The word *enthusiasm* comes from the ancient Greek meaning "Inspired by the gods." Any time you are enthusiastic, you are accessing godlike powers to enhance and bring vitality to your life, and to those around you. Yet many of us are often stingy with our enthusiasm, waiting for outside circumstances to *prove* to us that our enthusiasm is justified. Think of a person close to you, or a situation in which you have been withholding your enthusiasm. Find something—anything—you can be authentically enthusiastic about; give this enthusiasm openly and generously. Witness that person becoming empowered and starting to blossom. Then find the next thing and the next to be enthusiastic about. Be generous with your enthusiasm. Be inspired by the gods and experience the surge of wonderful vitality you'll be bringing into your life and the life of others.

TURNING THINGS AROUND WHEN THE GOING GETS ROUGH

My friend Jesse, an organizational consultant, is gifted in turning around multimillion-dollar companies that are on the verge of bankruptcy. I told him how I teach my clients to use enthusiasm to reach new levels of performance and vitality, and he exclaimed that this is exactly what he does for companies in trouble. He told me that when an organization is in a downward spiral and on the verge of closing its doors, people are still working very hard and expending lots of energy. However, the way they do it not only doesn't help, but it also often accelerates the downfall. People become fearful of losing their jobs. To make matters worse, there is uncertainty that deteriorates into suspicion, gossip, and blaming. This is a lower-level use of the brain that is very common when someone is under duress. Moreover, people tend to become entrenched in their habits and beliefs and keep on doing what isn't working.

Jesse tells the story of going into a large paper manufacturer, "where the *vultures* were circling," and discovering a great deal of distrust and animosity toward anyone coming in from the outside. During the first week, he visited the shipping department of the company, which he found to be the only department that was still functioning quite well. The team working there had been together for many years, had weathered many storms as the company went through several owners, and were generally optimistic that things would improve.

Jesse spent the afternoon observing the shipping operation, and by the time he stepped out into the parking lot to leave, it was getting dark. As he approached his car, several men made a circle around him. One of them was dangling a motorcycle chain from his hand and swinging it in a menacing way. The spokesman for this little gathering was one of the workers he'd met that afternoon. The group wanted to know what was going on and what Jesse's intentions were in terms of the company. They suspected him of being the "hatchet man" who would advise the present owners on possibly shutting the place down.

Jesse assured them that this was the furthest thing from his mind, that he, in fact, had been hired to advise management on changes that could be made to make the place profitable and stay open. He promised to meet with them in the plant the following day and give them a report on what he'd observed and what he was going to advise. At nine the following morning, he showed up at the shipping department, as promised, and set up a flip chart on which he'd prepared some graphs the previous evening. The workers gathered around and Jesse went through his presentation, showing what he thought was working in their department. He enthusiastically explained that their department was working better than any other in the company. Using his graphs, he showed why the shipping department was working so well, then asked the people around him to say more about what made their department tick. He would take this information to other departments and provide an infusion of new energy to upgrade their situation. Upon his departure from that meeting, he was escorted into the parking lot, but this time it was with much backslapping and handshaking. From that day forward, he was on a first-name basis with the men and women in shipping.

That day, Jesse helped the people working in the shipping department take a huge leap in upgrading their thinking and emotional organization. Moreover, he helped to create a model within the organization that he could refer to for guiding his work with the rest of the company. Jesse successfully turned the company around in a little under two years, and today it is one of the largest and most successful paper-manufacturing companies in the country.

When Jesse finished telling me the story, I realized that he had applied all the elements of enthusiasm every step of the way. He *paid close attention;* he *defined and named* what he and the company were dealing with; he *seized every opportunity* to help employees upgrade the quality of their own actions, and when things appeared negative, and even menacing, he stayed fully *committed* to turning the company around. He knew it was possible, *got into action, stayed focused* in the face of many setbacks and "impossibilities," *amplified* positive changes, including the small ones, focused on what was working, and *allowed for the miraculous.* In what people in organizational life considered record time, he turned the company around and got people performing in magnificent new ways.

Enthusiasm upgrades us and those around us and is a powerful way to bring about desired changes.

EXERCISE 5 ENTHUSIASM

WHAT'S YOUR VITALITY QUOTIENT?

On a scale of 1 to 5, rate yourself on each of the following statements, with 5 being always, 3 being occasionally, 1 being never.

1. When I am doing my exercise or fitness routine, I notice the smallest improvements and am thrilled by them.

2. I am able to generate enthusiasm for finding solutions in difficult situations.

3. I am able to generate enthusiasm when my child, spouse, or a friend does something I have asked of him or her, even when the outcome of his or her effort is not 100 percent successful.

4. I recognize when my energy gets dull and make sure to reawaken my enthusiasm.

5. I know enthusiasm to be real and see it as my responsibility to generate it consistently in every aspect of my life.

6. I find it easy to be enthusiastic when those close to me are successful.

7. There is nothing too small or too large for me to get enthusiastic about.

Score Yourself
24–35 points = high
15–23 points = medium
1–14 points = low

Go through the seven statements above and choose the ones on which you scored the lowest. Take some time to think about ways to improve your scores in those areas. The statements themselves will guide you.

Seven

Flexible Goals—Make the Impossible Possible

It is not the attainment of the goal that matters, it is the things that are met with by the way.

—HAVELOCK ELLIS

It's important to have goals in our lives. But we learn through NeuroMovement that the *way we pursue these goals* can either enhance or diminish our vitality. The *stuckness*, resistance to change, and being shut down that we sometimes associate with diminished vitality can be traced to the way we manage our goals. For example, the expression "Go for it!" implies that we should try to achieve our goals by the quickest route possible, *proving* to ourselves and others that we can go after what we want and get it immediately, if not sooner. Get rich quick! Find your soul mate in ten easy steps! Improve your sex life right now! Become an overnight success! We avoid anything that doesn't seem to directly contribute to getting what we want. But what promised to be a shortcut often isn't, leading instead to disappointment and discouragement. Vitality is diminished, which can kill enthusiasm for picking ourselves up and pursuing our goals in more enlightened ways.

Through Anat Baniel Method NeuroMovement we learn there really is a more enlightened way to set goals. We can accomplish more, with less suffering, and even open up to new possibilities by holding our goals loosely, approaching them with lots of flexibility. Those who do so reach much higher levels of accomplishment and enjoy greater, more sustained vitality along the way—even on those occasions when they never fully attain their original goals! Holding our goals loosely can seem indirect, wrong, off target, or too slow. But as you'll see, holding goals loosely, and having a flexible attitude while trying to reach your goals, is not only the surer way to succeed, but also an essential for vitality.

THE FIST IN THE ROCK

Goal setting is a powerful tool. It helps us get a lot of what we want from life—a vacation, a relationship, more money, better sex, a promotion, education, and so on. It also helps us through the tough challenges, such as earning a college degree, job training, getting through a family crisis, or setting up a budget to put money aside for a down payment on a home. If we're to succeed in achieving our goals, we have to be able to make intelligent choices about how to set them and how to go about accomplishing them.

However, most of us have been taught to pursue a goal by donning a set of internal blinders. Like the strips of leather worn by horses to prevent them from being distracted, our blinders sharply narrow our attention on what we believe we must do to achieve our goal. Sayings like "Keep your eyes on the prize" caution us not to be distracted by anything that doesn't appear to advance our ambitions. When we too rigidly focus on attaining our goals, we are less able to respond to feelings, experiences, information, or even new opportunities. We often overlook all consequences, including potentially undesirable ones, at times ignoring even our own well-being. In the documentary film *Animals Are Beautiful People,* there's a sequence that illustrates the consequence of focusing too single-mindedly on accomplishing a certain goal. The film shows how native hunters in the Kalahari Desert of Africa had devised a very clever way of locating water during the dry season. Through careful observation, probably over many generations, they discovered that baboons always had excellent caches of water that they carefully protected from other animals. It was almost impossible to track these animals to their watering holes since they were so careful to elude any possible interlopers.

To find the baboons' water, the hunters devised a way to get the animals to reveal where it was. The hunters first found a giant anthill, which baboons are known to frequent. These anthills, sometimes ten or twelve feet high, are made of hard, rock-like clay that has dried in the sun. The hunter makes a hole in the anthill just large enough for the baboon to reach into with a relaxed hand. Baboons, which are very curious creatures, will watch the hunter from a distance as he prepares this hole. The hunter then places some seeds within the hole, which he knows the baboons love to eat. Then the hunter goes off a ways to wait.

A baboon soon comes to investigate the hole and discovers the seeds inside. He wants them, so he reaches in, grabs the seeds, and clings to them with a tight fist. But now he cannot take his hand out of the hole; while the hole was large enough to slip a relaxed hand into, it is too small for the tight fist that now holds the seeds.

Not able to let go of the prize—the handful of seeds inside the hole—the baboon, in effect, traps himself. The hunter then approaches and the baboon goes into a panic, screaming in fear, somersaulting around the arm in the hole but unable to let go of the seeds, open his hand, and free himself. The hunter carefully loops a rope around the baboon's neck and gently takes the animal's free arm. It is only then that the baboon lets go of the seeds and removes his hand from the hole.

Now the hunter ties the baboon to a tree and gives him large chunks of salt to eat, a delicacy the hunter knows the baboon cannot resist. After eating the salt, the baboon becomes extremely thirsty. The hunter waits patiently until the next morning, all the while watching over the baboon's well-being so that it doesn't injure itself with the rope or become prey to another animal. By morning, the baboon's thirst is so compelling that he focuses on only one goal—to get to his watering hole.

The hunter now approaches the baboon carefully and frees it from its tether. The animal's singular goal of quenching its thirst takes precedence over everything else and it races off to the watering hole. Gone are his powerful instincts and skills for protecting the water. With one goal in mind, he acts without any consideration of the consequences of having someone follow him. The hunter is ready. As soon as the baboon takes off, the hunter is right behind, following the animal to the secret cavern where there is a pool of fresh water.

Sometimes we are so deeply invested in attaining our goals that we are like the baboon clinging to its prize. While we might not sacrifice our freedom for a handful of seeds, we might sacrifice our well-being and vitality for what might be described as a jaw-clenching approach to goals. An extreme example of this is found in the following story.

Some years ago, the Chicago Columbus Day marathon was called off because temperatures were reaching into the nineties and humidity was over 90 percent. Not exactly the best weather for a long run! Even when dozens of people started collapsing, thousands of others kept running. Hundreds of people ignored the extreme discomfort of their own bodies and continued the race until they required medical attention. The authorities, with the recommendation of doctors, had to stop the remaining runners and force them to disperse. Sadly, one man in his thirties died. The intense emotional attachment to achieving the goal of the marathon led thousands to ignore their well-being and safety, putting their health and their lives at risk.

This story epitomizes jaw-clenching goal setting at its worse. Our obsession with physical fitness has led to overtraining and training injuries that are epidemic, even among schoolchildren. We reach for goals and expect to attain them right away, as if our bodies and brains were capable of attaining highly demanding feats and refined skills without taking the time to figure them out and work up to them gradually. This problem has become so widespread that treating injuries due to poor training has become a billion-dollar industry.

In our everyday lives, it can be all too easy to lose sight of the price paid for our rigid approach to goals. For example, a young couple, recently married, shares the worthy goal of having a nice house, fine furnishings, and a new car. They both have good jobs, so they take out a big mortgage and get the house, the furnishings, and the car of their dreams. Soon they realize that paying their mortgage and other loans is requiring them to work so hard that they barely get time to see each other, their stress level increases, and their vitality plummets.

Or consider the woman who, on the first date, asks the man she's with how many children he wants to have when he marries. Ouch! She has the poor guy contemplating parenthood with her even before finding out whether they like each other. His reaction is to withdraw and end the evening early, and never to call her again. The young woman later tells her best friend that she only wanted some assurances that this was a relationship worth pursuing. Nevertheless, by putting her goal so far ahead of the process of getting to know her date, she ruined any possibility of the relationship developing.

We even carry our rigid approach to goal setting into raising our children. For example, we do it when we attempt to keep our children on track through high school, to prepare them for getting into a good college. With our internal blinders set in place and our attention focused and narrowed, we dedicate time, money, and personal energy into guiding our children toward the right credits that will get them into the college of their choice. We watch them knuckle under, attending class, studying, and working to achieve the best grades. The sad thing is that by following this rigid process, many children get turned off education. Their time is so rationed and sparse that they dare not study or do hardly anything except what is deemed useful for achieving their goal. There's less and less time for socializing, for exploration and discovery of what's interesting for them, or for enjoying leisurely activities with family and friends. Many top colleges are now observing that while today's freshmen are test-wise and academically accomplished, they lack the ability to think for themselves or explore "outside the box."

Even if we are not causing major injuries, driving away our dates, getting bogged down with mortgages, or deadening our children's intellectual curiosity, ignoring the necessary process to achieve our goals may produce just the opposite of what we are seeking. Instead of feeling vital and energetic, we end up feeling sore, discouraged, and weary. Our lack of knowledge about how to achieve our goals often leads us to give up on desires and personal objectives that otherwise are quite within our capacities—in all areas of our lives. Being savvy about the process of achieving our goals is not only the best way to avoid injuries and disappointments, but it also ensures higher levels of accomplishment, greater mental, physical, and emotional well-being, and certainly higher levels of vitality.

EXERCISE 1   UNINTENDED CONSEQUENCES

Think of a time when you went after a goal with your blinders on. Nothing was there for you except the goal and the finish line. And, ultimately, you were successful at achieving that goal. Looking back on that experience, did achieving this goal also result in any undesirable consequences you hadn't anticipated? For example, did you end up with an injury to your body or tension in an important relationship? Were there any undesirable consequences that overshadowed your accomplishment of that goal? In what ways did these affect your sense of well-being, your vitality, or the enjoyment of your success? In your mind, can you imagine going after the same goal with your blinders off, gaining the freedom to see more of what was going on along the way, which might have led to different choices? Would some of those undesirable consequences have lessened while still accomplishing your goal? Had these consequences been lessened, how would this have affected your vitality?

ARE WE SMARTER THAN BABOONS?

The baboon in our earlier example clings to the seeds even in the face of serious threat to its well-being—being captured by the hunter. And later, the goal of quenching its thirst overrides the need to protect its water. Once the pattern of grabbing the seeds is activated in its brain, the animal has no choice but to go through with it. This is not unlike what happens when we set a goal, become intensely attached to attaining it, and then establish a specific pattern of behavior for achieving it. We repeat the same pattern, clinging to it with a tight fist, trapping ourselves, regardless of the outcome. We can get so emotionally attached to a desired outcome, and so locked into a repetitious pattern, that we really can't see anything else, allow for the new, or imagine there is any other way to achieve our goals. This fist-in-the-rock approach to our goals renders us incapable of making any real choices along the way. At such times, we generate repetitive brain activity that doesn't leave much room for invention, discovery, change, and evolution.

In his award-winning book *Ever Since Darwin,* Stephen Jay Gould explores human qualities that have evolved over the millennia, some of which distinguish us from all other creatures. As he points out, "We are preeminently a learning animal. We are not particularly strong, swift, or well designed, nor do we reproduce rapidly. Our evolutionary advantage lies with our brain, with its remarkable capacity for learning by experience." We are not like other animals who are hardwired to develop their most mature and powerful abilities within a few days or weeks of their birth, like the cheetah, which is designed to run at seventy miles per hour, or the honeybee, which instinctively gathers nectar.

We humans, unlike more-instinct-driven creatures whose very survival depends on rapid maturity, are designed to develop slowly, processing billions of pieces of information, gathering, synthesizing, refining, and creating. We do not depend on fast-maturing capacities but rather on the unique, evolving, open, and ongoing integration of information. We owe the gifts of our extraordinary accomplishments to our brain's need to grow and change through the influx of new experiences and information. At birth, our brains are roughly a quarter of their adult size. They continue to grow at rapid rates, forming trillions of new connections that not only help us survive, but also enable us to create and reach capacities that otherwise wouldn't be possible. From this, we might be wise to take a cue: For us to thrive in the way nature has designed us, we need ample time to immerse ourselves in the full process of living instead of driving blindly toward a goal.

When we are inflexible in our approach to a goal, it can be as limiting as being stuck in a rut. There is little opportunity for our brains to innovate. Play leads to discovery, feeding our brains with information to create new and unexpected possibilities. As Patrick Bateson, the noted biologist, said, "Play is the best way to reach certain goals." Through play, we can avoid what he called "the lure of 'false endpoints,' a problem-solving style more typical of harried adults than playful youngsters." He adds that by "noodling away at a problem we might well arrive at something better than the first solution." When we hold our goals loosely, we give our brains, our bodies, and our minds the space they need to change, grow, and correct the course of action when necessary. This is our best insurance not only for success in achieving our goals, but also in avoiding injuries, getting ourselves too deeply in debt, or taking on more than we can handle. Instead, we are able to respond to the present, where our brains best perform their creative magic.

Holding goals loosely, the young couple from our earlier example might have put off tying themselves to a large mortgage, giving them more time, with less pressure, to enjoy each other, develop their relationship, and have more freedom for other endeavors. The single woman, by simply taking genuine interest in her date, might have discovered that he was lots of fun and thus developed a friendship that would enrich both their lives in unexpected ways. And had the high school kids been less pressured to "perform" academically, they would have had the opportunity to explore their own interests and develop more creative thinking.

Our greatest accomplishments often arise unexpectedly, sometimes with results that surpass our aspirations, when we remain *in the process,* that is, flexible and allowing for the new to form or appear. Being in the process in this way is the mine of our richest treasures and the source of our greatness. What arises from this process, whether it is the fulfillment of our stated goal or a complete surprise, feeds us and spurs our vitality. Some of the most creative musicians, artists, and scientists have experienced the benefits of allowing time and patience, with room to explore and play. Wolfgang Amadeus Mozart once reflected:

> When I am, as it were, completely myself, entirely alone, and of good cheer—say, traveling in a carriage, or walking after a good meal, or during the night when I cannot sleep; it is on such occasions that ideas flow best and most abundantly. Whence and how they come, I know not; nor can I force them.

The human brain has extraordinary powers for discovering what is needed and for innovating solutions to meet those needs. And it is often these unexpected solutions that make our lives so interesting and dynamic. The joy and exhilaration a small child feels as she learns to say her first word or take her first step or run for the first time comes from her free, unattached participation in the process of discovery and the accomplishment of these new skills she didn't even know she was about to realize. Once she does, she feels powerful, energized, somehow knowing that her achievements have come from herself. She is ready to move on to the next thing. When we hold our goals loosely as adults, we recreate this early life experience for ourselves, with joy and exhilaration as we progress toward achieving our goals.

EXERCISE 2 UNEXPECTED FREEDOM

With the following NeuroMovement exercise, you'll experience freer hip joints by holding that goal loosely.

PREPARATION

Wear comfortable, loose-fitting clothes that will not restrict the movements you are about to do. Have a thin cushion, mat, or simply a soft carpet to sit on. Do the exercise with your shoes off, with warm socks if you like. Make certain you will not be interrupted for approximately fifteen minutes.

THE EXERCISE

1. Sit on the floor, bend your knees, and open your legs to the sides with the soles of your feet touching. Place your hands on the floor behind you so that you can lean on them comfortably. Look at your knees and note how close or far they are from the floor. You might notice that one of your knees is closer to the floor than the other. Bring your hands forward and—*gently please!*—push down on the insides of your knees as you to try to bring them closer to the floor. Let go and see if this made any difference. Most likely not.

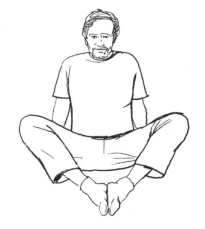

2. Lie on your back with your arms at your sides. Bend your knees, open your legs to the side, and put the soles of your feet together as before. Feel how your pelvis contacts the floor. Now pull your belly in—contract your abdomen muscles—rounding your back and rolling your pelvis up a bit. You will feel your lower back pressing more into the floor and your tailbone lifting a bit off the floor. Now stop and let go of your belly muscles, allowing your pelvis to roll back down. Do this movement slowly back and forth six to eight times

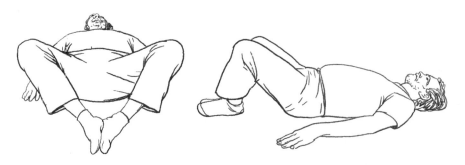

Each time you do this movement, feel how your knees tend to move away from the floor when you pull your belly in and move closer to the floor when you let go of your belly. Stop. Slowly lengthen your legs to rest for a moment. Feel how your body is lying on the floor.

3. Lie on your back again with your knees bent out to the sides and the soles of your feet touching each other. This time, slowly and gently arch your lower back and roll your pelvis downward so that your lower back moves away from the floor and the pressure moves to your tail-bone. Make sure to *push your belly out* as you arch your back and roll the pelvis down in this way. Then come back to the middle.

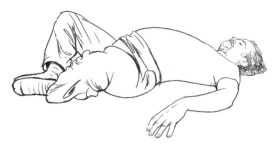

Repeat this movement six to eight times, slowly and comfortably. Can you feel that each time you roll your pelvis down, your knees open to the sides a bit more?

Stop, bring your legs down and rest for a moment. Feel how your body is contacting the floor. Do any parts of your body begin touching the floor more fully?

4. On your back, resume the same position with your legs and the soles of your feet and this time combine the two movements—pull in your belly and roll your pelvis up, then arch your back, push your belly out, and roll your pelvis down. Rock your pelvis back and forth in a continuous movement four or five times. Rest, straighten your legs, and feel how you are lying on the floor. Can you feel any further changes in the contact your body has with the floor? Are you breathing differently than before, more fully?

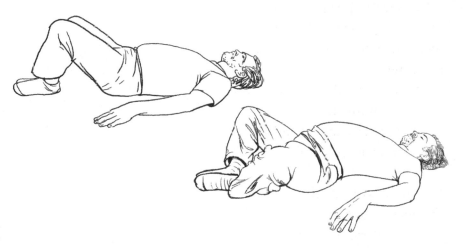

5. Lie on your back with your knees to the sides and the soles of the feet together. This time, arch only the left side of your lower back and roll your pelvis to the right, moving the pressure to your right hip. Your right knee will now come a bit closer to the floor. Make sure to do the movement with your back and pelvis, not by lifting your left knee up to the ceiling. Each time you do the movement, think of pushing your belly out to the right. Do the movement four or five times. Stop and rest for a moment.

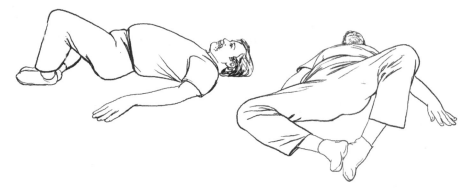

6. Lie flat on your back with your knees to the sides and the soles of your feet together, this time arching the right side of your lower back only and roll your pelvis to the left to move the pressure onto your left hip so that your left knee comes closer to the floor. Make sure to do the movement with your back and pelvis, not by lifting your right knee up to the ceiling. Each time you do this movement, make sure to push your belly out to the left as you do the movement. Do the movement four or five times.

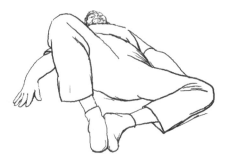

Stop, extend your legs, and rest for a moment. Notice if there are any other changes in the way you feel or lie on the floor.

7. Lie on your back with your knees to the sides and the soles of the feet together. Combine the two movements above, rocking your pelvis right and left with one knee coming closer to the floor than the other. Do a light, easy movement, back and forth, five or six times.

Stop, extend your legs, and rest for a moment.

8. Lie on your back with your knees to the sides and the soles of the feet together. Resume the movements you did in step 4, rolling the pelvis up and down and pulling the belly in, then pushing it out. Is the movement any different than before? Is it any easier, with larger, smoother range? Do your knees open sideways more than a few minutes ago?

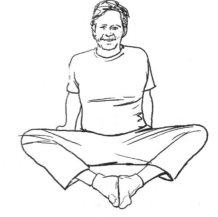

9. Sit once again with the soles of your feet touching, your knees out sideways, leaning on your hands behind you as you did in the beginning of this exercise. Roll your pelvis forward, push your belly out, and look at your knees. Are they closer to the floor then before?

Get up on your feet and just stand for a moment. Notice if you feel different than usual. You might feel taller, maybe lighter, or more grounded. Now walk around. Do your hips feel freer? Is there a bit more bounce and life in your step?

THE HUMAN WAY OF ACHIEVING GOALS

Abraham Maslow, a leading psychological researcher, explored what goes on inside us when we are most deeply and fully and authentically engaged in our lives, enjoying whatever activity involves us. In his book *The Farther Reaches of Human Nature*, Maslow said that hard-line, linear goal setting can rob us of the "joy in life that makes it worth living." He believed that rigid goal setting makes it impossible for people to experience the "all-too-few moments of total life-affirmation which we call peak experiences." He put great emphasis on leaving room in all our endeavors for self-discovery. It is here that we identify what we're about—our values, what brings us pleasure, our innate potentials and abilities. We then learn how to apply these in the discovery of activities that provide us, on an ongoing basis, with vitality, joy, and well-being.

The model of goal setting that Maslow describes parallels a natural process of self-discovery and evolution that we go through as small children, leading us to enormous accomplishments in those early years. As discussed earlier, we have our greatest growth and rate of accomplishment during the first five years of our lives. But it's worth noting that during this period, we are operating without conscious goal setting, without a timetable, and are accomplishing a huge amount. Children delight in the experience of their newfound abilities—what Maslow calls *the joy of self-affirmation*. NeuroMovement helps to bring this awareness into our adult lives on a daily basis.

We know from studying the lives of very successful people that there is another piece to the puzzle, a capacity of the brain that allows us to hold to a chosen goal while simultaneously responding to infinite possibilities. It can both take in new information from the outside and generate new possibilities from the inside. The human brain is unique in its ability to create new pathways and possibilities, to find creative and novel solutions, and to carry out those new possibilities even under duress. The American novelist F. Scott Fitzgerald was observing this when he said, "The test of a first- rate intelligence is the ability to hold two opposed ideas in the mind at the same time, and still retain the ability to function."

Our brains have the capacity to operate both within very rigid, limited, and automatic patterns and within elevated, open, and flexible patterns wherein we can work vigorously toward a goal, all the while being wholly aware and responsive to both inner and outer stimuli and opportunities. When we are able to operate in this way, we can change course with great ease and flexibility to match what is called for in the moment. We have what I call a "re-versible approach" to our goal; we can change course in creative ways on our greatly unpredictable path to achieving our goals. For-get controlling the outcome! Our brains have the opportunity to create evolved and complex patterns that give us solutions we couldn't have planned for in advance or rushed into. Pursuing our goals in this way is a great boost to our sense of power and vitality.

The tendency to approach our goals with a tight fist is very common. Under duress, we tend to regress and act in the compulsive and automatic ways we saw in the baboon example. However, we are all quite capable of upgrading our brains and developing a flexible and responsive approach to achieving our goals.

We don't know for sure whether we could train monkeys to open their hands and release themselves from the hole in the rock when they are threatened. However, we need not get our proverbial fists caught in the rock anymore. We can approach goals with elevated creativity and innovation to enjoy greater vitality and higher energy.

STEPS FOR HOLDING GOALS LOOSELY

Here are twelve steps that will guide you in holding your goals loosely, ensuring higher levels of accomplishment; greater mental, physical, and emotional well-being; and certainly higher levels of vitality. This is the NeuroMovement process for setting goals.

1. IDENTIFY. Name and describe in some detail something that you want and don't currently have, or a way that you want to be, or an outcome that you would like to bring about. A goal is wanting to create something that is not there yet.

2. CREATE A PROCESS. Remember that achieving your goal is a process and that you play an active role in it. Know that the process will take an undisclosed amount of time, unless your goal is extremely simple and immediate for you, perhaps something that you already know how to do and that does not call for a change. Take your time; allow your brain the opportunity to feel, create, investigate, and invent.

3. WONDER. Remember, until you reach your goal, you cannot know exactly how you will get there or what the experience of achieving that goal will be. As you continue on your path, practice

wondering how your path will unfold, always leaving room for the new to occur. In this way, you will avoid falling back on existing rigid patterns of behavior.

4. **BACK OFF.** Always put process ahead of outcome. Rushing to achieve the outcome, trying to reach too far ahead of yourself, often creates discomfort or injury. If you try too hard, too fast, too big, or too soon, you risk learning limitations that may lead you to give up before you accomplish your goal—and will deplete you of energy and vitality.

5. **PLAY.** On the way to your new accomplishment, be like a child: Play; let your path meander in different directions in what might seem like a waste of time. Know that each time you take on a goal, small or large, you step into the unknown. Your brain will thrive with all the new information it gets, all the while discovering new possibilities for you, some of which might catapult you toward your goal in unexpected ways.

6. **BE FLEXIBLE.** As your path unfolds, you might want to adjust your goal, or perhaps change it altogether. So many great breakthroughs were discovered on the way to seeking something else.

7. **FINE-TUNE.** Make the goal truly yours. Fine-tune it as you progress toward the goal, always asking if this is what you really want. Do it with large goals, such as what you want in your relationships or your career. Also do it with simple goals, such as choosing what you want for dinner or what you might like to do after work.

8. **LET GO.** Do not try to control the outcome. When we try to control the outcome, things begin to go awry. The brain needs freedom to create and integrate billions of bits of information; this is how we form the new. This is impossible for the brain to do

when we try to control the outcome. When we are willful and rigid about the outcome, we are presuming to know what we do not yet know and are stuck with re-creating what we already have.

9. INTEND AND CHOOSE. Replace your natural tendency to want to control the outcome. Instead, bring your attention to the process. In this way, you gain the ability to choose what to do and how to do it at any given moment, and you discover your own unique path to achieving your goal. With your hand open rather than tight-fisted, you gain access to the vast resources of your brain. This is also when you are filled with vitality, power, and vigor, feeling and setting into motion your full aliveness.

10. BE WRONG. Allow yourself lots of *mistakes*. Embrace mistakes. Do not worry about doing it *right*. Mistakes create a treasure trove of information and opportunity for your brain and yourself to discover a way to achieve your goal. Our brains are not prewired to do what we do. Instead, we are self-correcting systems that require lots of experimentation in order to have all we need to achieve our goals. The greater and more challenging the goal, the more room we need for mistakes and self-corrections. When we fear mistakes, we drain the life energy from the process and risk achieving only lesser goals or giving up altogether.

11. APPLY REVERSIBILITY. Keep a loose, open-ended attitude toward your goals. At all times, make sure that you can imagine yourself achieving your goal or failing to achieve it with the same ease. See yourself getting what you want—or not—with the same degree of comfort. This is when your brain is operating at a high level, able to move in any direction and create new, unexpected, and remarkable possibilities. You then pull in the full richness of who you are. You are open, allowing greater resources not just from yourself but also from the universe around you to contribute to and transform your process for getting there.

12. **BE FREE.** Ask yourself, who's running the show? Are you making the best use of your *human advantage,* taking your time to explore and discover? Or is your automatic, fear-based, unconscious self—the tight-fisted brain and person—controlling your choices and actions? Embrace your human advantage.

DELIGHT IN THE PROCESS

Back in my early years of studying with Dr. Moshe Feldenkrais, I began working with a child who had Down syndrome. This was the first child that I'd ever worked with. After the first session, I realized that I had no idea what to do. I immediately turned to Dr. Feldenkrais for help. After I described the child to Moshe, he showed me a number of things I could do to try to help the child. The next time the mother brought the child to a session, I did what Dr. Feldenkrais suggested, and it worked like magic. The child stayed focused and interested in everything I did throughout the session. I was ecstatic. I felt that I had arrived—that I knew what to do.

When the boy returned the next day, I began working with him as I'd done the day before, expecting the same kind of magic. To my surprise, while it was not catastrophic, the session didn't work nearly as well as the day before. The child was squirming and obviously not nearly as interested or involved. I was crushed. Just twenty-four hours before, I had thought I had it nailed . . . but now? I called Moshe on the phone and said, "There is no question that you are the most amazing genius, but what about me?" I continued, "When I followed your guidance, it was like magic, but once that ran out, I was back at square one."

"Anat," he said, "you have to make a choice between being a good technician or growing to become like a world-class artist."

He explained that I would become one or the other depending on the attitude with which I approached my goals. If I went for getting the outcome right here and now, the best I'd ever do would be to become a decent technician. If I wanted to become a Jascha Heifetz, he said, a practitioner of the highest quality, and be able to reach the highest levels, I would have to do things very differently.

He then shared a story with me about when he was a student of physics earning his Ph.D. with Frédéric Joliot-Curie at the Radium Institute in Paris. They were working with radioactive material that was extremely dangerous if you came into direct contact with it. He told me to think of picking up a glass of water and pouring some of it into another glass. While this was a simple task with water, it posed very serious health hazards with the radioactive liquid they were working with. To go forward with their research, they had to develop techniques for safely handling containers of radioactive liquid while pouring precise amounts into test tubes. It took over a year to figure it out. A "go-for-it" approach to their goals at that time, such as simply picking up a radioactive container with their bare hands, could have cost them their lives. While developing the technology for handling radioactive material might have seemed like a detour to some people, it turned out to be an important achievement in itself, one that opened the way to remarkable discoveries for future atomic research.

Dr. Feldenkrais concluded that if I wanted to be a Jascha Heifetz, a true artist of my trade, with all the thrill, interest, energy, and creativity that comes with it, I needed to develop a *reversible* relationship to my goals. This meant that I should place little importance, at any given moment, on whether I achieved my goal. Instead, I needed to throw the goal into the distant future like a gentle light that would guide me, and at the same time turn my focus and interest on the process, free to follow any detour that was required. When I hung up the phone after our talk, I felt calm and available to focus on the child, the process, and on any resource, internal or external, that might provide me with ideas and solutions for how to proceed. I knew I had been handed an enormous gift by my teacher.

People who enjoy high levels of vitality know, either consciously or unconsciously, that their continued vitality comes from a very different source than from succeeding or failing to achieve a specific goal. Certainly, there is satisfaction in attaining one's goals, just as there is disappointment in not attaining them. Vitality lives *in the process itself*, and that means embracing all that comes along, be it the expected or the unexpected—living in the now.

Exercise 3 Ready, Set, Play

For this exercise, choose a simple goal that you care about but about which you don't feel the world is going to stop if you don't achieve it. Playfully think of *at least three different ways* you might accomplish this goal. For example, you have a huge bunch of cut flowers of varied colors and want to arrange them around the house to brighten things up. Play with different possibilities for arranging them. Spread them out on a table and randomly pick up individual flowers, putting them with others to discover new combinations of color or type.

Let's say you're helping your child learn spelling or math. Or perhaps you are helping a fellow employee learn a new office procedure. Look for ways to be playful. Make deliberate mistakes that he will catch; you may well find that this wakes up his brain and gets him to understand faster than if you rigidly insisted on his doing the task correctly from the start. Focus on the learning process while holding the goal lightly. Be creative and experiment, bringing real vitality into the moment. If you do, the outcome will take care of itself.

Some of the things that you try might not work. Remember, that is perfectly fine. Play with making errors. For example, if you're learning a new software program at home or at work, don't load important data at first. Instead, try different things with the program, even if it leads to a mistake. You'll learn a great deal about the program's potential and how to correct errors, and you'll reduce your own anxiety about what might happen if you push the wrong button.

Continue doing this exercise for a week with as many small goals as you can think of. As soon as you feel you have gotten good at holding goals loosely and coming up with different ways for achieving them, start applying this process to larger and more challenging goals you have set for yourself. Experience the sense of freedom, joy, and vitality that comes with approaching your goals this way.

DON'T LET SUCCESS DULL YOUR VITALITY

It's easy to understand how failure can stop us and dull our vitality. What people often don't realize is that success can have a similar effect, and often does. Olympic gold medalists, for example, often tell how after winning the gold they go home, and when the excitement and congratulations of friends, family members, and the media subside, they suddenly experience a terrible letdown, sometimes followed by depression and a lack of interest in life. After the successful achievement of a goal that has demanded so much of their lives, many winners have described their victories as ultimately feeling like a door had been slammed in their face.

We see the same pattern in virtually every area of life, especially where people have worked hard to achieve important goals. In a recent *New York Times* article, author Gary Rivlin profiled Max Levchin, who in 1998, at the age of twenty-seven, created the online payment service called PayPal, later sold to eBay. eBay paid $1.5 billion for it, of which Levchin received $100 million. Levchin said that the year following the sale was the worst year of his life. He spent the best part of that time, he told the reporter, "feeling worthless and stupid," baffled by the thought of what he was going to do with the rest of his life. He even considered returning to college to earn a doctorate degree. Even though he possesses a fortune, he is back to spending most of his time creating a new start-up company.

We humans are blessed with a slow, protracted period of development that keeps the learning process open-ended for longer than any other species. As Stephen Jay Gould claims in his book *Ever Since Darwin*, the marked slowing down of our development, and the growth of our brains, has provided us with opportunities to evolve way beyond any other creature, and to achieve what no others have. When we take our time and keep the process of working toward our goals open-ended, we give ourselves and our brains exponentially more options for growth. We gain a huge advantage by doing the same with every goal we have. The key is this: *Do not try to close the deal too soon. Do not make crossing the finish line your primary goal.* We are built to take our time. It is when we are most ingenious that we are most alive—and most successful at achieving our goals.

Recently, Nobel Prize winner Oliver Smithies, a geneticist, was interviewed by Christopher Lee of the *Washington Post*. Smithies stated that winning the Nobel Prize was completely unexpected but "very gratifying." He added, "My work was never toward getting the Nobel Prize, it was solving a problem and enjoying the solution."

EXERCISE 4   HOLDING GOALS LOOSELY

WHAT'S YOUR VITALITY QUOTIENT?

On a scale of 1 to 5, rate yourself on each of the following statements, with 5 being always, 3 being occasionally, 1 being never.

1. I like having goals in my life.

2. I am intentional in the ways I go about achieving my goals.

3. When I take an exercise class, or am playing at sports, I enjoy being in the process even if I haven't yet reached my goals.

4. When making plans with other people, I find that "getting off course" is interesting and often an opportunity for something better than I expected to occur.

5. When helping others, I make sure to be playful, welcoming mistakes as an important part of the process.

6. In whatever goal I might have, I realize I do not know ahead of time exactly how it would be accomplished, but I do know it is possible if I keep all venues open.

7. When pursuing my goals, I quickly become aware of any unintended negative consequences and change my course.

Score Yourself
24–35 points = high
15–23 points = medium
1–14 points = low

Go through the seven statements above and choose the ones on which you scored the lowest. Take some time to think about ways to improve your scores in those areas. The statements themselves will guide you.

Eight

Imagination and Dreams— Create *Your* Life

Imagination is everything. It is the preview of life's coming attractions.

—ALBERT EINSTEIN

The dreamer and his dream are the same . . . the powers personified in a dream are those that move the world.

—JOSEPH CAMPBELL

Our brains have the capacity to dream and to create from within ourselves, as if out of nothing, something that is new. Through NeuroMovement we learn to use our ability to daydream, envision, and imagine to fuel our vitality. The degree to which we are able to dream and imagine will determine not only the life path we follow, but also the vitality and personal power we experience around everything we do, from the most fundamental skill to the goals we may choose for ourselves later in our adult lives.

When you dream and imagine, lights turn on throughout your brain, creating billions of new neurological connections. This ability to form new connections through imagination and dreaming is our ultimate human gift, allowing us to move beyond our limitations and rigid old habits, creating new possibilities and realities that were not possible for us before.

Our creative and imaginative powers are intensely alive and active as children. We reach out into the world, developing new skills and abilities, and we become increasingly aware of the seemingly endless possibilities around us. We see another child riding a bicycle and imagine ourselves doing that, too. Instantly, our brains are forming new connections at a furious rate. Unbeknownst to us, our capacity to imagine and dream moves us into doing something we couldn't do before, filling us with energy and vitality. Unfortunately, by the time we reach adulthood, most of us have stopped using our dream and imagination faculties, at least to some extent.

Daydreams allow us to explore endless possibilities in the safety of our minds. They may take us to exotic lands, or allow us to experience ourselves in ways we never have before—heroic, funny, brilliant, accomplished, loving, or wealthy. It allows us to feel how it might be to live in a beautiful house, or to brave the challenges of climbing a mountain, or to be an astronaut flying to some distant planet. Daydreams also reveal our authentic selves, and our true passions.

When we develop ways of giving our dreams expression in the real world, we tap into a limitless wellspring of energy and passion. Guided from within and directed by our dreams, we make choices that empower us, filling us with passion and enthusiasm. We are able to accomplish what otherwise would have been impossible. Connecting with your dreams and living your life from your authentic self is essential for achieving your greatest vitality. And you'll soon discover that knowing and following your dreams doesn't just energize you, but also inspires those around you.

Dreaming—a Rich and Fertile Ground

Most people believe that our minds are usually focused and clear, paying close attention to whatever we are doing, only daydreaming during idle, unguarded moments. We may even have negative associations with daydreaming, for instance, that only very unproductive and lazy people engage in it. In recent years, however, science has uncovered a much different picture of daydreaming.

In a study of how our brains operate during normal day-to-day activities, Dr. Malia F. Mason and a team of researchers found that while psychologists have traditionally "assumed that we spend most of our time engaged in goal-directed thought and that, every so often, we have blips of irrelevant thoughts that pop up on the radar," the truth is that "most of the time we are engaged in less directed, unintended thought and that this state is routinely interrupted by periods of goal-directed thought."

Mason's research was conducted using functional magnetic resonance imaging (fMRI) to observe activity within the brains of their subjects when they were engaged in activities that required high levels of mental concentration, then compared them to times when they were daydreaming. One of the conclusions of this work was that there is a default network in our brains associated with daydreaming. The fMRI scans showed that this default section really lit up, revealing a great amount of activity whenever subjects began to daydream.

Moreover, the fMRI scans showed that the default network of our brains involves not just one but a wide variety of regions, including lobes that are in charge of impulse control, judgment, language, memory, motor function, problem solving, sexual behavior, socialization, spontaneity, and the processing of sensory information. In other words, our brains come to life—*they light up*—when we dream.

In another study of six thousand men and women, Steven Jay Lynn, a psychologist at Ohio University, and Judith Rhue, a psychologist at the University of Toledo, found that creativity, problem solving, and empathy were stronger in those who fantasized than in those who did not fantasize. Their brains were constantly creating new information that might be applied to problem solving or a broad perspective of issues at some future time. The researchers also concluded that those who fantasize (daydream) are far more interesting, flexible, spontaneous, and creative than those who do not. Let's not forget that what makes people interesting is that they themselves lead interesting and vital lives, presumably a product of their abilities to create new information and new patterns in their brains.

What these studies suggest is not only that it is normal and healthy to daydream, but also that when we are daydreaming, we may very well be integrating information, organizing it, and creating new connections for later application in our lives. *Daydreaming is a fertile state that allows our brains enormous flexibility to pull together unpredictable solutions and inventions.*

A variety of research involving dreamtime during sleep suggests very strongly that the benefits of daydreaming also occur during sleep. During what's called REM (rapid eye movement) sleep, when we are most actively dreaming, our brains are mixing, matching, and juggling traces of information, often making connections that perhaps we would not make in a waking state or when we are more focused and goal oriented. The experiences of our lives, stored as memory, are pulled apart and put back together in new or different order. Information is shuffled and reshuffled, making new connections. Often this produces dreams of situations that would be impossible, or certainly bizarre and unlikely, in our everyday lives. All of this is rich fodder for creativity, problem solving, and a highly flexible, interesting, and constantly renewing view of our lives. Think of it as generating vitality.

The dream state—whether waking or sleeping—is the source of inspiration, even as it is integrating thoughts, images, and ideas. Matthew Wilson, a researcher at the Massachusetts Institute of Technology, states that during sleep, different areas of our brains talk to each other, asking for and receiving the latest information that we have gathered during our most recent experiences during the waking state. Dr. Wilson speculates that this process is similar to what goes on in our minds when we take a moment, free of distractions, to reflect, perhaps daydream, and sort out the meaning of events we've experienced during the day, replaying them in our minds, creating alternatives to what actually happened, and flagging important details for future reference. According to Dr. Wilson, there is no question that dreaming is an essential process. Rather than confining ourselves to a limited repertory of existing patterns, dreaming offers us new possibilities, a wellspring of vitality. Allow yourself to dream.

EXERCISE 1   TAKE A DAYDREAM BREAK

When is the last time you recall daydreaming? Next time you feel a bit stuck, depleted of energy, perhaps feeling somewhat hopeless about something in your life, take a few minutes for a daydreaming break and let your mind wander. Perhaps create a lovely story for yourself and discover what new possibilities you come up with. If you haven't daydreamed for a long time, you might find that your first daydreams seem a bit dull or mundane. Keep at it, embellishing your daydreams and using your creativity to create daydreams that really delight you. If you find yourself in any way inhibiting yourself, such as telling yourself that what you are daydreaming about couldn't possibly happen, go ahead and dream your "impossible" daydream anyway. Remember, you are in charge of creating your own daydreams. Feel your hesitation or doubt and do it anyway. Daydreams awaken your brain to create new possibilities for your life, and this becomes a powerful source of vitality.

THE POWER OF IMAGINATION

The brain's innate capacity for dreaming is expressed in both voluntary and involuntary ways. Whereas dreaming seems to bubble up from within our minds, it can be thought of as *involuntary;*

imagination—the godchild of the dreaming brain—which is often more conscious and deliberate, can be thought of as *voluntary.* Imagination is an integral part of any process of change, be it making plans for a trip to Hawaii or drawing up the blueprints for a new house. It is integral to any new reality that is in the process of being born. Imagination is invaluable for creating the new, vitalizing both our inner and outer worlds.

Thanks to your imagination, you have the ability to upgrade the quality of your brain's functioning, creating new pathways and inventing new and refined ways of moving, thinking, and feeling. In research conducted by Alvaro Pascual-Leone, two groups of people were taught to play a simple five-finger exercise on the piano. After learning the exercise, the first group practiced these exercises for five days by moving their fingers accordingly. The second group mentally practiced the exercise—using only their imaginations. Unlike the first group, they did not move their fingers at all. At the end of the five-day period, as one would suspect, areas of the brain associated with doing the exercise for the first group grew. What researchers also found was that the changes in the brains of the second group were the *same* as the first group. Imagination is real, and it has a measurable impact on our brains. The Pascual-Leone study concluded that mental practice "seems to place the subjects at an advantage for further skill learning with minimal physical practice." Developing our imagination skills gives us greater mental powers and physical capabilities.

To demonstrate the power of NeuroMovement in my seminars, I have students lie on their mats and do an exercise that is limited to one side of their bodies; then I have them imagine doing the same exercise on the opposite side of their bodies. Initially, most people find it more difficult to imagine the movement than to actually do it. After a few moments, I have them compare how the two sides of their bodies feel, based on freedom of movement, strength, precision, and the pleasure they experience as they move about. They soon discover that the outcome for the side they have *imagined* moving in the exercise often feels and moves better than the side they actually exercised. The movements on the imagined side are smoother, stronger, more precise, better coordinated, and more pleasurable.

EXERCISE 2   IMAGINE!

The following NeuroMovement exercise is an immediate way to experience how imagination can create new patterns in our brains. In this exercise, we will do a common movement, one that you will already be fa-miliar with. Try this quick exercise and experience in your own body how your movement, guided by imagination, can change and improve. You may then call up the power of your imagination and utilize it intentionally to make desired changes in your every-day activities.

PREPARATION

Create a time and a place in which you have approximately five or so minutes to yourself, with no interruptions. Work with a mat or other firm but comfortable surface, preferably on the floor, where you have plenty of space. Wear loose clothing that won't restrict your movements. Be barefooted or in your stocking feet.

THE EXERCISE

I. **INITIAL POSITION.** Lie on your left side with your right leg and foot on top of your left leg and foot. As the drawing shows, bend your legs at the hips and your knees about ninety degrees, or as you find comfortable. Extend your left arm above your head, palm up or down, whichever is more comfortable for you, and rest your head on your upper arm. (*Note:* This will be what I'll refer to as the *neutral position* in the rest of the instructions.) Extend your right arm out in front of you, straight at the elbow, and rest your hand gently, palm down, on the floor, directly out from your shoulder.

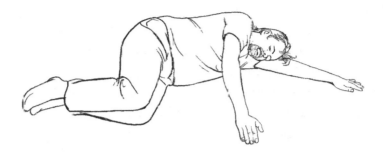

2. ACTUALLY MOVING. Lift your right arm slowly and gently toward the ceiling and bring it back to your neutral position, that is, palm down on the floor. Lift your arm again toward the ceiling. As you move it, make sure you see and follow your right hand the whole way, moving your head to the right to keep the hand in sight. If it is easy to do, continue moving your arm in the direction of the floor behind you. Make sure to keep your right knee and right foot on top of your left knee and foot, and go only as far as you find comfortable. Then come back to the neutral position. Twist your upper body gently to accommodate this movement. Do this movement four or five times.

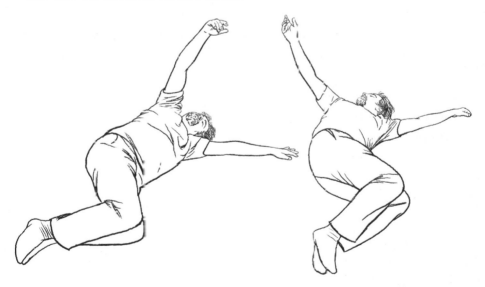

3. IMAGINING MOVING. Make sure to read the following instructions all the way through, at least once or twice, before doing them.

Lie on your left side and resume the neutral position from the previous instructions. From now on, you will be imagining yourself doing the movements, but you will not actually be moving your body. Instead, imagine you are lifting your right arm toward the ceiling and behind you, seeing your hand the whole time as you did in the previous instructions. Now, as you imagine doing this movement, also imagine the whole length of your spine as a chain that is twisting as you raise your right arm. In your imagination, bring back your right arm to the front and untwist your spine. Repeat these movements in your imagination three or four times.

Continue imagining the same movements of the arm, seeing and following your hand the whole time. Just this time, imagine your rib cage getting very free and the spaces between your ribs expanding—like a fan that is opening—as you twist your back and move your arm around. In your imagination, come back to neutral and repeat this movement three or four times. Next, imagine the same movement, and this time think of your sternum— your chest bone—moving to the right as your right arm lifts and your body twists around. Repeat this in your imagination three or four times.

Now, once again imagine lifting your arm, following your hand with your eyes and head as before. This time imagine your spine, ribs, and sternum all at once. Imagine the movement to be very easy and pleasurable to do. Repeat three or four times.

4. ACTUALLY MOVING. Go back to actually doing the movement and see if it has changed. Is it easier to do? At the same time, are you moving farther than before?

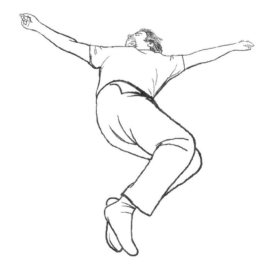

It's Harder to Imagine Than to Do

Students and clients often ask me why it is more difficult to imagine doing a movement than to actually do it. For a moment, imagine that I ask you to raise your right arm toward the ceiling. Your response will probably be pretty immediate. You'll reach up and in a split second your arm is pointing straight at the ceiling. The chances are that you have done this movement thousands of times, and you will do it all very automatically, probably without giving it a second thought. All the myriad of messages, to and from your brain, that guide the trajectory of this movement are *grooved*, that is, they are following patterns that you created a long time ago and have followed for many years, perhaps for most of your life.

What happens when we are called upon to imagine that movement—and I mean imagine it in minute detail—is that we no longer automatically follow all those messages to and from our brain, guiding us, every tiny fraction of an inch along the way, as to how far, how fast, and how much energy to put into the movement. We no longer depend on the old groove to guide us. When we imagine, we have the opportunity to create new and different ways of doing—in this example, reaching toward the ceiling. Really imagining a movement like this means not just seeing the movement of our arm in great detail, but also feeling it, and even imagining the slight rustling sounds of our clothes as we imagine doing the movement.

When you are imagining the movement and no longer depend on the old patterns and grooves that carry the information to lift your arm, you provide your brain with the opportunity to work at a much higher level and invent new ways and solutions. Out of such moments come the feelings we associate with vitality—surprise, playfulness, the excitement of new discoveries. You are also creating new information for your brain, information that it can use for upgrading the patterns to lift that arm in the *future*.

Many years ago, when my father was in his late fifties, he

attended one of my classes, in which he was by far the oldest participant. I introduced the class to a new, very challenging sequence of movements. None of the participants were able to do the movements, regardless of how hard they tried. It was obvious to me that the way they were trying to do it was not going to work. While the class was struggling to accomplish the movements, I noticed that my father lay very still on his mat, with his eyes closed.

After several minutes, while the rest of the class was still struggling, I watched in amazement as my father executed the sequence of movements with such incredible ease and perfection that it took my breath away. When he had completed the movements, he lay back on his mat to rest, with a look of deep satisfaction on his face. I, however, was not going to let him get off quite so easily. I had the class turn its attention to him and asked him to do it again. He paused, returning to his previous state of focus and concentration. Then, as the entire class watched, he did it again. For a moment you could have heard a pin drop in the classroom, then came a sigh of deep amazement that sounded like it was shared by everyone in the room.

A young woman in the class, a dancer, asked with astonishment how it was possible that she, trained in movement, could not do what my father, more than twice her age, was able to do with such ease and grace. The answer my father gave that day revealed not only how he had done it, but also how the dancer, too, could do it.

My father told us, very matter-of-factly, that he initially tried doing the movement a couple of times, and it became clear to him he was not going to succeed. He then decided to try something he'd done in the past. Instead of struggling, he stopped moving his body; instead, he imagined his skeleton doing the movement. He explained that when he imagined himself as just a skeleton, stripped of his muscles and skin, he could then imagine the trajectory of the movements, and they became effortless and clear in his mind. Once he was able to imagine the entire movement that I'd assigned, from beginning to end, in spite of it being rather challenging, he did the exercise *in the flesh*, as it were, and it was very easy to do.

My father had never done those movements before that moment. Through imagination, however, he was able to upgrade his brain to perform the complex new series of movements.

INVISIBLE POWERS THAT PROMOTE VITALITY

You can feel the benefits of applying your imagination in any area of your life. It might be an interaction with a loved one, the way you deal with your boss, what kind of lover you will be, or how you will manage your money. Imagination is one of the most powerful tools for upgrading your brain, and your experience of life, in a conscious and deliberate way; NeuroMovement gives us that way.

To increase and maintain vitality, it is important to experience the power of imagination firsthand and to understand that it is *real*. We tend to look upon anything that we can't immediately see, touch, taste, smell, or hear as "unreal." We tend to earmark anything that's physically intangible as "made up" and of little consequence. Nuclear scientists, however, have changed all that, demonstrating over and over again that much of what goes on in the universe is invisible to the naked eye as well as to our other senses. While we can't always see the presence of something through direct observation, we can know it's there by its impact on the environment around it. For example, if we're indoors looking out on a windy day, we cannot see the wind itself. But we can observe its presence in the sway of the trees, or the flurries of leaves that it lifts and blows about on a fall day. And we may also be able to hear it howling around the eaves.

The *invisible*, or imaginative, made possible by the human capacity for dreaming, can and does impact our lives in significant ways—intellectually, emotionally, and physically. In an interesting study published in *Psychological Science*, Alia J. Crum and Ellen J. Langer worked with a group of eighty-four female room attendants employed in seven different hotels. The researchers divided their subjects into two groups: The first, called the "informed group," was told that the work they did, cleaning hotel rooms, was good exercise and that it satisfied the surgeon general's recommendations for an active lifestyle. They were shown examples of how their work provided the right exercise. The uninformed group was told nothing. Neither group changed the actual work they were doing.

After four weeks, the two groups were examined for exercise and health considerations, and their results were compared with the examinations they received at the start of the test period. It was found that the informed group showed a "decrease in weight, blood pressure, body fat, waist-to-hip ratio, and body mass index." The uninformed group had no significant changes.

Note here that there was only one difference between these two groups during the monthlong period of this study: Only the informed group was told that what they were doing provided the proper exercise to meet the surgeon general's recommendation for an active lifestyle. In other words, their imaginations brought about measurable physical changes. Applying imagination, with its upgraded brain energy, can transform the outcome of anything we might do.

EXERCISE 3 IMAGINE!

NEW POSSIBILITIES

One of the areas in which we tend to be most challenged is in our emotional reactions to events around us. So often our emotional patterns are deeply grooved; they seem to take over, hijacking us, before we even know what's happening. Imagination is a great way to invent new patterns of response. With our ability to imagine, we can mentally and emotionally rehearse our encounter with a difficult person or situation, first away from the actual situation, then by bringing the newly created patterns into action in real life.

Think of a person in your life with whom you often have a difficult time. You may find that this is someone with whom you seem to have the same emotional reaction, behaving in ways you want to change. It might be with your child, your partner, a neighbor, an employer, or a friend. Vividly re-create the situation in your imagination, with as much detail as you can. Include details such as what the person looks like, and the sights, sounds, and colors of the place where the difficult encounter might take place.

Think about the location, the sound of your voice and the other person's voice, the words you expect to hear, and the thoughts, feelings, and emotions you normally experience. Once you have re-created the scene clearly, begin to introduce changes in your imagination. Invent new thoughts, and begin to experience new feelings and emotions. Remember that you are totally in charge here. This is all taking place in your imagination, so you can have it anyway you wish.

Repeat this exercise as many times as necessary, until you have a whole new set of possibilities of what you think, how you feel, and how you act in your imagination. Then get yourself into the actual situation. Keep the first encounter brief while implementing a few of your newfound possibilities. Gradually increase periods of exposure to the difficult situation, always making use of all the new patterns and reactions you have been creating in your imagination. Over a period of time, you will find that your new patterns are replacing old ways of acting and responding. The new patterns are becoming grooved and you are gaining new freedom, freed of unwanted patterns that once controlled you.

We consume a huge amount of energy with old behaviors and feelings that no longer serve us and which, in fact, cause us a good deal of difficulty. By addressing these old patterns in the way described, we free energy to be used in more creative ways and gain vitality that might otherwise be inaccessible to us.

Imagination—Building Your Skills

We are all born with a built-in capacity to imagine. In our childhood, we use imagination spontaneously. Then, in adulthood, we tend to inhibit our imagination. That doesn't mean it's gone. But if we're to enjoy vitality, we need to reawaken our imagination. It's helpful to remember that imagination is a skill, and like any other skill it requires intentional use and practice if we want to get good at it and reap its maximum benefits.

In Marty Klein's book *Beyond Orgasm,* the author talks about the use of what he calls "mental rehearsal" and other mental imagery techniques for enhancing sexual pleasure with our partners. For example, the use of imagination can be employed to help women who have difficulty achieving orgasm with their partners. Women who'd had traumatic sexual experiences early in their lives may have painful memories that numb them, preventing them from experiencing any kind of sexual pleasure. They can reclaim their sexual pleasure by first paying attention to when these old, painful memories come up. Then they deliberately initiate fantasies of pleasure that allow them to respond to their own and their partner's pleasure. Over time, as they master new skills in the use of their imaginations, they are able to enjoy intense and satisfying orgasms with their partners.

Imagination may be part of our birthright, but we vitalize its full promise only through intention and practice. With practice, you will increasingly appreciate why imagination is real and how you can use it to make significant changes in your life, transforming the ways you may presently be doing things, moving past struggle and pain into more freedom, inventiveness, and joy in everyday living.

The following nine steps will help you improve both your imagination and your vitality.

- **ACKNOWLEDGE**. Recognize that imagination is real.
- **CHOOSE**. Make a conscious decision to develop imagination and begin applying it intentionally in your life.
- **SELECT**. Decide on an area in your life that you would like to improve or enrich, or in which you would like to have a breakthrough. This might be in a relationship with a family

member or friend, or in your work. It could be in your sex life, or something to do with your leisure time, your money, your health, and so on.

• **FOCUS.** Turn your attention to one of the areas you have selected to improve and find an aspect of it that is comfortable for you to think about.

• **DAYDREAM.** Take some time to let your mind meander around your area of focus. Give yourself the luxury of daydreaming. Let your thoughts and feelings drift freely, exploring and inventing whatever might come up around your area of focus.

• **BE AN OBSERVER.** No matter what you come up with, even if it is unpleasant, outrageous, or seemingly impossible, do not censor it; just observe it. View it as a resource—raw information that is neither right nor wrong, good or bad, unless it is acted upon. Remember that imagination is a powerful tool. Keep daydreaming until you come up with something you like and that will likely enhance you and those around you.

• **EMPOWER YOUR HIGHEST SELF.** Choose from your daydreaming those parts that you feel and think will be most useful, positive, and beneficial to yourself and others.

• **MENTALLY REHEARSE.** Take the parts you selected from your daydreaming and in your imagination apply them in that specific area of your life you would like to improve or enrich, or in which you would like to have a breakthrough. Remember that since this is your own imagination, you can make sure that everything you envision will be easy, comfortable, safe, and successful. Be sure to include in your mental rehearsal other people and the impact of your imaginary actions on them.

• **GIVE IT A TRY.** Once you feel satisfied with your mental rehearsal, go ahead and try it out in action. See how well you like it. If it is not working as well as you'd like it to, go back and daydream and imagine some more. If you like the outcome, go on to the next area you would like to enrich, improve, or have a breakthrough in.

As you develop these skills and incorporate them into your life, your increased creativity and inventiveness will make it possible for you to do things in new and better ways. You will begin experiencing the miraculous more often.

"I Have a Dream . . ."

Most of us have heard the famous speech of Martin Luther King Jr. in which he announced to the world, in powerful tones, "I have a dream that one day on the red hills of Georgia the sons of former slaves and the sons of former slave owners will be able to sit down together at the table of brotherhood." In that speech, he articulated a vision that guided his own life and the lives of millions of people. It stirred the hearts and minds of people the world over. Most assuredly, it stirred the hearts and minds of anyone who shared the belief that apartheid and racism are wrong.

Not all visions, of course, move nations or even, for that matter, are shared by people other than the person who has created the vision and perhaps the people closest to him or her. What we recognize in Martin Luther King Jr.'s example is the power of a personal dream to focus our lives, providing a high level of coherence that organizes our brains and thus the choices that guide our lives. What we know about King's vision is that his dream came out of his deepest and most personal beliefs and experiences.

Don't worry if your dream for your life seems modest. For most of us, the dreams and visions that inform us are very personal and private, highly individualized, and critically important if we're to live healthy lives. I am recalling an incident that happened many years ago in a workshop given by Dr. Feldenkrais. He had asked for a volunteer to demonstrate his work. A number of people in the class raised their hands, and he pointed to a woman who moments later struggled to the front of the room supported by an aluminum walker. When Dr. Feldenkrais asked her to tell him what her life's dream was, the woman, Felicia, was quick to explain that she had cerebral palsy. Ever since childhood, and throughout the forty-five years of her life, her dream had been to walk independently, without the clumsy walker she had to push around.

After her lesson with Dr. Feldenkrais, Felicia stood up, first with his help and then without, and within moments she was walking on her own. Everyone was moved. Then, as she was returning to her place, without the walker, Dr. Feldenkrais called her back. She turned around and looked at him quizzically. He told her there was something very important they needed to take care of now that her dream had been fulfilled. He explained that while she had fulfilled her dream of being able to walk independently, that gift could end up diminishing her well-being, or even turn into a curse, if she failed to take the time to create a new dream for her life. The two of them sat down, and he patiently counseled with her as she discovered and defined her next dream.

EXERCISE 4   YOUR DREAM BOARD

A mystic once said, "The best way to predict the future is to invent it." Jack Canfield, the cocreator of *Chicken Soup for the Soul*, tells how he has done just that. He describes how he created a "vision board" that he hung on his office wall. He attributes the realization of his dream—the sales of millions and millions of copies of his books—in great part to this *dream board*.

Select a dream you may already be manifesting, create a new dream, or refresh an old one in the following way: This can be a small dream or a very large one; just make very sure it is *your* dream. Get illustration board for your dream board at any art supply store. It comes in a large selections of sizes, from fifteen by twenty inches on up. You then want to collect photos, or images cut from newspapers, magazines, or off the Internet that represent different parts of your dream. Fasten these to your board with tape, tacks, or glue.

Update your board regularly, refining your vision as you go

along. Jack Canfield recommends sitting in front of this dream board at least once a day to constantly feed your brain with these images that represent your dream.

IT HAS TO BE YOUR DREAM

If most of us are not compelled, as Martin Luther King Jr. was, to change the world, it still matters that our dream comes from our own inner source. There's a wonderful quote from the classic novel *Doctor Zhivago*, by Boris Pasternak, that helps to spell out the importance of following our dream:

> Your health is bound to be affected if, day after day, you say the opposite of what you feel, if you grovel before what you dislike and rejoice at what brings you nothing but misfortune. Our nervous system isn't just a fiction, it's a part of our physical body, and our soul exists in space and is inside us, like the teeth in our mouth. It can't be forever violated with impunity.

Joseph Campbell, who coined the phrase "follow your bliss," understood the potency of getting in touch with our most personal and innermost dreams. He spoke of this process as the "ultimate adventure" of our lives, one that becomes possible when we "embrace our own personal destiny" by trusting and being guided by what we love. In their book *Take This Job and Love It,* Dennis Jaffe and Cynthia Scott said:

> People who follow a dream or have a deep sense of purpose about their work are rewarded with an almost inexhaustible supply of energy. People moved by this internal energy source are fired up by inspiration. They are likely to find the energy required to finish the difficult, even mundane tasks that go into any achievement.

Where this type of dream comes from is a mystery. But we do know that our brains construct it out of what we were born with and the infinite numbers of experiences and possibilities that make us who we are. Discovering and following these dreams is the path to high levels of vitality and energy at any age. Bestselling author Gary Zukav calls it our "authentic power," and states that it is about "doing what you are supposed to be doing. It is fulfilling. Your life is filled with meaning and purpose . . . You are happy to be alive."

So many people, famous and not so famous, have reiterated this same idea. It is what Einstein was referring to when he said that "the gift of fantasy has meant more to me than any talent for abstract, positive thinking." And it is what Henry David Thoreau was reflecting on when he said, "If one advances confidently in the direction of his dreams, and endeavors to live the life which he has imagined, he will meet with success unexpected in common hours."

Abraham Maslow saw these visions and dreams in a similar light: "Authentic selfhood can be defined in part as having the ability to hear these impulse-voices within oneself, i.e., to know what one really wants or doesn't want, what one is fit for, etc." This reminds me of something my teacher, Dr. Feldenkrais, often said: "Our health and ultimate vitality come out of our ability to realize our dreams—our known and declared dreams, our undeclared dreams, and even those dreams still hidden from us." Each and every one of us needs to have a dream if we're to thrive.

You've Got to Have a Dream

You may have heard the words of the song from the musical *South Pacific*, by Oscar Hammerstein and Richard Rodgers: "You gotta have a dream. If you don't have a dream, how you gonna make a dream come true?" Our dreams call to us from our future. They organize our brains and provide the wind under our wings that lift us to our greatest heights of vitality. And if there is anything that diminishes our vitality, it is this: *not having a dream.*

FRAN CAME TO ME with complaints of lower back pain that her medical doctor had told her was stress related. He was concerned, however, that if she didn't get help, her problem could become more serious, possibly requiring surgery. Fran lived halfway across the country, but her daughter, who lived near me, knew of my work and thought it might help. During a visit with her daughter, Fran made an appointment with me.

The first thing I noticed when Fran walked into my office was that she walked with a slight stoop and shuffled her feet, which made her appear to be at least twenty years older than she really was. During our initial interview, I learned that while Fran's doctor had given her a clean bill of health in every other way, he had written her a prescription for pain pills and antidepressants. She did not want to take the pills, but she was still considering doing so because she was finding both the back pain and the emotional pain unbearable. Meanwhile, her daughters were worried because Fran had become increasingly reclusive over the past few months.

During Fran's first session with me, I immediately saw that her energy was extremely low and her voice expressed little or no vitality, even when she was talking about her first grandchild, Stacey, who had been born within the past year. Five years before her grandchild's birth, she told me, her life could not have been more perfect. She and her husband, Thomas, had raised two beautiful children, both now grown and on their own. They had also built a very successful gardening and nursery business in the small town where they'd lived. Thomas and she had looked forward to retiring in eight years, traveling to Europe, where they'd never been, and enjoying time with their growing family. Thomas, however, was diagnosed with cancer, and after three years of difficult treatment, and a long period in a nursing home, he finally succumbed to the disease.

Fran had been devastated. All the dreams she had shared with her husband, she said, were destroyed; with Thomas's death, she felt that her life, too, had come to an end. She confessed that she no longer found any purpose or meaning in anything she did. She had great employees who were very supportive, helping her keep the family business going. But the truth was that she cared very little even about that. She showed up for work less and less, only calling in from time to time to see if there was anything that required her attention. I asked her how she felt about her new grandchild. She said that while she found joy in spending time with the baby, and holding her, it also made her very sad when she was reminded that Thomas had not lived long enough to share this happiness with her. He had looked forward to becoming a grandfather.

As I worked with Fran employing NeuroMovement techniques, her pain began diminishing and she talked about dreams she and her husband had shared. I asked her if she could envision herself creating a new dream, one for herself, a dream that could perhaps also capture some of the things she and her husband had enjoyed together. We discussed how it needed to be a dream that would bring pleasure into her present life without Thomas. I explained to her that our dreams are like road maps that guide us in our lives and into our futures. Without dreams that have a very deep and personal meaning for us, rising from within our own being, it is easy to lose all interest in life. For sure, I told her, we can have no vitality, no *joie de vivre* without a dream.

For the first time since I'd met her, I detected a little smile and maybe even a little sparkle in her eyes. Yes, she told me, before he became ill, she and Thomas had drawn up plans to create a sanctuary garden on a piece of property owned by the church where they were members. When Thomas became ill, they had had to put this project on a back burner, and until this moment she had forgotten about it.

I pointed out that this would not only be a great dream to pursue, but that it would also be a wonderful way to express her love for her husband and all that they had shared in their life together.

Within weeks, Fran was fully engaged in the dream of creating a beautiful sanctuary garden. She seemed to change overnight. A few months after our last meeting, I received an invitation to a groundbreaking celebration for the garden, which was to be dedicated to the memory of her deceased husband. When I saw Fran again, some months later, she was like a different person, full of energy and enthusiasm, intensely interested in life, and living it to the fullest. Her dream has evolved in the years since so that she is now designing personal sanctuary gardens for private residences, and has made quite a name for herself.

Our dreams not only organize our brains, and our lives, but they help to determine the depth of our engagement with life. It is the depth of our engagement and action that provides us with opportunities for creating, achieving, and connecting with others in ways that allow us to feel profound satisfaction within ourselves. Dreams are elusive, since in themselves they have no tangible form. At least in the beginning, they exist only as swirls of interacting brain cells. But if you view them as the beginning of form, and look around you to see that everything created by humans began in this way, you will appreciate their power even more.

Our brains function at a very high level when we dream and use our imagination. Dreams and imagination are, if you will, a demonstration of negative entropy—that is, the increased quality of organization and functioning in the brain. They counteract the natural and constant tendency toward entropy—the loss of order and reduction in the quality of whatever we do. With minute amounts of energy in our brains, we create visions that organize our actions and simultaneously attract energies around us that contribute to manifesting our vision.

Often, all that's required to restore our vitality is to look carefully at what's happened to our dreams. Fran's story clearly illustrates this process and how it can play out in real life. When her husband died, the dreams she had shared with him died with him. If she wished to go on and enjoy a vibrant, purposeful life again, she had to find within herself the material for the new dream that called to her from her future. Without a future, it's as if we fall into a dark pit of hopelessness. The best we can do is shuffle through our lives like automatons.

We need not suffer a crisis, or great loss as Fran did, to lose the vitality our dreams once provided. On the contrary, sometimes it happens as a result of fulfilling our dreams. For example, in our twenties, we might have the dream of getting a good job, owning a particular kind of car, getting married, and having our own home. For six or seven years, we know exactly what we want, and we have a huge amount of energy for getting it. At some point, we achieve our dreams or we come close enough. We have the house, the car, the marriage, and the job. Life seems complete and whole. But then things begin to shift. We no long feel called by the future. The dream we have dreamed for most of our adult life is behind us because we've attained that dream. As a student of mine, a young man in his thirties, put it, "Whatever force it was urging me forward was gone. The plug had been pulled and my motor was winding down." Being in the process of fulfilling our dream heightens our vitality. Once our dream has been fulfilled, or is no longer our true dream, we need to go on to create another.

ACTION MAKES DREAMS COME TRUE

Dreams have a magical quality. But let's not get seduced by the idea that the magic will take care of itself. Dreams require action, real work, courage, persistence, and intention for them to materialize. I am thinking right now of a man whose story illustrates this point very clearly. His son told me how his father, Dale, very early in his life had decided to become an electrical engineer. He spent sixteen years with one company and worked his way into a top management position. Then the company he worked for was bought out and he was let go.

He was at first crushed by what had happened. He had seen himself as working for another eight years for this company and then taking an early retirement. Now he was looking at starting all over again with a new employer. He went to a headhunter in search of another job, but after looking at several positions, he became more discouraged than ever. He realized that what he'd been doing was no longer his dream. He didn't want to go back to what he'd been doing for sixteen years. A close friend of his advised that he take time off, get away from the city for a while, and look to find his future path.

Dale took a couple trips with his family, read a lot, and spent evenings in his home workshop, where he pursued his hobby, which was woodworking. One night, he finished a project he was working on and brought it into the house to show his wife. As he proudly showed off his handiwork, he casually remarked that as he was working on this piece he realized he was following his heart's desire. This was what he wanted to do for the rest of his life. He beamed happily as he said this. His wife nodded enthusiastically. Why not? she asked. Perhaps he should explore this possibility. At first, he rejected the idea. He was certain he couldn't make a living that way. Besides, he was trained to be an electrical engineer, not a woodworker. The upshot of Dale's story was that he in fact did abandon his first profession and followed the dream of becoming a woodworker. Dale and his wife sold their house, simplified their lives, and for a time lived on their savings and her income. Dale was giving birth to a new dream that he reported was far more compelling than the first. After four years of hard work, he had established a line of high-end custom furniture that was in great demand.

His son told me that these were happy years for the entire family.

Realizing our dreams takes work. It also takes courage and persistence. The dreams that guide our lives are always in the process of growing and evolving. Even as we get to know what these dreams are about—and what we ourselves are about—one dream can cease to provide what I've described here as the call from our future and cause us to lose all vitality. We need to watch out that what began as our dream, giving us powerful direction and vitality, doesn't become routine and dull. If our dream is no longer appropriate and meaningful to us, we need to be aware of this and create a new dream.

Exercise 5   Dream Action Plan

Dreams are powerful in themselves, but they are exponentially more powerful as you couple them with action. Jack Canfield did not stop with the dream board. Every day, he took two or three actions, any actions he could think of, to help move his dream forward. Take the dream you have selected in the previous exercise (see page 223) and every day come up with at least three actions that match your dream. This will energize you and the universe to make your dream a reality. The action might be a phone call, an e-mail you send, a class you take, a product you create—the list is endless.

Dreams Are a Precious Resource

Our capacity to dream is a powerful resource, one that is unique to human beings. It is out of this capacity that we have probed the secrets of the universe, analyzed the human psyche, and developed amazing capacities for healing. It is the source of all art and science. Our personal dreams guide our everyday lives and direct our actions in such a way as to make it possible for those dreams to be fulfilled. Yet as powerful and essential as our dreams are, they are also fragile and vulnerable, and we must protect, nourish, and love them just as we would protect, nourish, and love a small child. Our dreams give rise to new possibilities, out of which has come a constant flow of new inventions and innovations from tens of thousands of years. In spite of the fact that humanity has created untold millions of new inventions, and successfully challenged the limits defined by conventional wisdom, skeptics flourish, ready to proclaim the impossibility of whatever new ideas are being put forth.

On October 9, 1903, for example, the *New York Times* published the following: "The flying machine which will really fly might be evolved by the combined and continuous efforts of mathematicians and mechanicians in from one million to ten million years." On that same day, at Kill Devil Hills, North Carolina, a bicycle mechanic by the name of Orville Wright wrote in his diary, "We unpacked rest of goods for new machine." On December 17 of that same year, just two months and a week later, the Wright brothers' flying machine made its first successful flight.

It seems we are never without a shortage of skeptics and naysayers. Eight years before the *New York Times* article, Lord Kelvin, a British mathematician and physicist, and member of the British Royal Society, proclaimed that heavier-than-air flight was simply an impossibility. Not only did two lowly bicycle mechanics prove him wrong, but sixty years later humans would fly beyond Earth's atmosphere and land on the Moon.

Had the Wright brothers, and all the millions of others whose dreams have shaped history, listened to their skeptics and naysayers, or taken their critics to heart, we would still be living in caves and hunting food with pointed sticks. It is important to remember the endless possibilities of which the dreaming brain is capable and to understand that we can make those possibilities real.

Exercise 6 Create!

WHAT'S YOUR VITALITY QUOTIENT?

On a scale of 1 to 5, rate yourself on each of the following statements, with 5 being always, 3 being occasionally, 1 being never.

1. I find myself daydreaming from time to time and enjoy it.

2. Whenever confronted with problems or challenges, I use imagination to seek solutions.

3. I see imagination as real and encourage it in myself and others.

4. I agree with Einstein that "imagination is more important than knowledge. Knowledge is limited. Imagination encircles the world."

5. Visions and dreams of others frequently inspire me.

6. I make sure to always create and hold a dream—big or small—for myself and my life.

7. I take action to make my dreams come true.

Score Yourself
24–35 points = high
15–23 points = medium
1–14 points = low

Go through the seven statements above and choose the ones on which you scored the lowest. Take some time to think about ways to improve your scores in those areas. The statements themselves will guide you.

Nine

Awareness—Thrive with True Knowledge

For every man the world is as fresh as it was at the first day, and as full of untold novelties for him who has the eyes to see them.

—ALDOUS HUXLEY

One of the oldest and most universal teachings throughout the ages has to do with self-knowledge. As far back as the eighth century BC, the following words were inscribed over the entrance to the Oracle at Delphi, whose council was sought during difficult times: "Know Thyself." We find the same wisdom expressed in the work of great spiritual teachers such as the Dalai Lama and Mahatma Gandhi. They advocate self-knowledge as the foundation of human happiness, effectiveness, love, peacefulness, and vitality.

There cannot be self-knowledge without awareness. As far as we can tell, the capacity for self-knowledge—to know ourselves—and knowledge of others and of the world around us is uniquely human. This amazing capacity is made possible by our ability to observe our own thoughts, feelings, and actions, as well as our ability to observe the world around us and to know that we are observing them.

Awareness is different from attention, which we've explored in some detail in earlier chapters. Attention is when we focus on something, be it in our environment or in ourselves. But it is possible to pay attention without being aware that we are doing so. Think of yourself listening to a friend telling you a captivating story. You are extremely interested, fully focused and attentive to her, perhaps even "carried away" by the story she is telling. You might or might not be aware at that moment, however, that you are totally wrapped up in your friend's story. You may not be aware of the expressions on your face, your breathing, or your feelings and thoughts. We see this frequently with young children when they are fully attentive to something they are observing or doing, to the exclusion of everything else. It is a very common experience in all of our lives to be giving our full attention to an event or action and at the same time have little or no awareness of ourselves or our environment.

Awareness, as I use the term here, means *knowing that you know, knowing what it is you know, and even knowing when you don't know.* You are aware that you raised your voice, or that you are pleased with something your boss said to you, or that you are ticked off at something your spouse said. If you make a mistake while cooking a special meal, you know that you've made that mistake, and you know you can choose to correct it. When moving your body, you know that you are moving; you know where you are and what you're doing. You are aware of your thoughts and feelings, and can even observe yourself being aware. Awareness makes it possible for us to know what's going on around us, and to recognize the impact of our thoughts, feelings, and actions on ourselves and others. All this can be realized with NeuroMovement.

Your level of vitality is directly related to your level of awareness. By increasing your level of awareness, you will be able to act with increasing precision, variety, efficiency, and creativity, as well as gaining greater freedom of thought and feeling. Other animals have some rudimentary consciousness, of course, but little or no capacity to observe and be aware of themselves. Without consciousness, they would not even be able to seek the basic necessities of life. Dogs recognize what's to come as their master starts packing up bags to take yet another trip. When a flock of geese fly in formation, they know when to relieve their leader and have another goose take its place in the front of the V. The human capacity for awareness, however, is extraordinary, far above anything we have found in any other life-form. The tools and knowledge of NeuroMovement expand our capacities for more fully realizing our awareness, thus expanding the opportunities for the greater energy, enjoyment and vitality that await us.

We reap the benefits of awareness every day of our lives. When we are in a heated exchange with a friend or coworker, awareness lets us know when things are going awry, giving us the freedom to change course and work toward a satisfying experience for both of us. When jogging or working out at the gym, our awareness allows us to recognize movements that strain our bodies, providing an opportunity to look for more beneficial ways of doing those movements. We become aware of certain ways of communicating with a loved one that works well for him or her and we make sure to use it in the future. Our awareness of stress gives us a chance to calm down and work more efficiently while putting less strain on our bodies and minds. And think how awareness gives caring parents the ability to seek ways of guiding their children's behavior that are empowering for that child.

Without awareness, we would be slaves to our habits, bound by automatic behaviors that we have learned in the past; it is through awareness that we not only know what we are doing at any given moment, being fully in the present, but awareness also makes it possible for us to transcend our present way of being. It is at the heart of improving our individual lives and evolving human awareness in general. Without awareness of self and others, we are left with few means for being anything but reactive and, ultimately, victims of our circumstances.

Following the limiting routines of a life without awareness, we would be missing our brains' incredible capacities not only for forming new connections, but also for upgrading itself to a higher level of functioning, and would soon be worn down by life. As humans, we are not endowed with instincts such as those of most other animals; rather, we depend on our awareness of ourselves and our relationships with the world to guide us. Awareness offers us the ability to observe and know ourselves, to observe the world around us, and to create alternatives that can improve the quality of our lives and the lives around us. Our awareness, made possible through our observational capacities, is tantamount to our ability to function successfully and be truly vital.

AWARENESS TRUMPS AUTOMATICITY

The observer self is when we are *present in the moment*, bringing our full awareness to the *now*. It is more than just "seeing" or "noticing" what's going on around us. Perceiving a stimulus and even reacting to it does not mean that we are aware of it at all. Think of someone driving a car, deeply involved in a conversation with another person, yet able to stop when a signal turns red, or follow changing conditions of the road. Awareness—knowing, and knowing what we know—requires a different activity and organization in the brain than does attention alone. Awareness changes us. Through awareness, whatever happens to us becomes part of us. Without awareness, we could move our hand, for example, thousands of times and nothing new would be happening in our brains or our bodies. Without awareness we could do something new and it would be as if it never happened. With NeuroMovement we explore, discover and expand this miraculous capacity for awareness, and are changed forever.

One of the things most astounding about awareness is the lack of it. We can live with certain habits and automatic responses to life that to an outside observer might appear incredibly obvious, but not to us. We acquired these habits unaware, and we are so accustomed to them that they are invisible to us. They have become like the air we breathe. Whether those automatic behaviors serve us well or not, we have no choice but to repeat them, over and over again. Yet no matter how long we have had an automatic response, once we become aware of it, knowledge rushes in, and the transformation of that response begins. This growing awareness is the opening for new options, bringing about movement and change, creating a shift in us that allows us to experience our lives in new ways that are more fun, lively, creative, and effective. It is so powerful that awareness in one person can bring about a shift in another person close to him or her, sometimes producing a domino effect, changing a whole family, work environment, or community.

Gail, a tennis coach for young children, attended an evening presentation during which I introduced two of the Nine Essentials: *variation* and *holding goals loosely*. I led the group through a short movement lesson, during which they experienced the power of applying these essentials to transform their movements and achieve freedom and flexibility many of them did not previously have. A week later, I got an e-mail from Gail telling me about four boys she had been coaching. Born quadruplets and premature, these boys had some challenges. For a year, Gail had been unable to get them to do an overhead serve.

Gail explained to me that during my presentation she had become aware of her belief that she had to push her students to achieve goals she'd set out for them and "drill" them with endless repetition. Once she became aware of her belief—self-knowledge— she completely changed what she was doing with the boys. Instead of telling them to "try harder" to do the serve correctly, she began introducing a number of different variations, many of which appeared to have nothing to do with developing the overhead serve. She did not tell the boys what she wanted them to accomplish. That way, she made sure they would not get stuck on trying to achieve what they had been failing to achieve for a year. By the end of that first hour, all four boys were doing the overhead serve easily.

In another example, Ronda, a psychotherapist and artist in her late forties, had always been interested in personal evolution and growth. She was a faithful yoga student and meditator. She was no newcomer to awareness. In one of my weekly evening classes, I introduced the group to the idea that we do not have a "neck" like we have an arm, a leg, or a head. It looks like we do because it is that part that pops out above our shoulders. I told the group what we really have is *one long spine and that the top part pops out.* Instead of thinking of the neck and spine as separate when we turn our head or bend it or lift it, I asked them to become aware of the whole spine (from the sacrum to the base of their skull) as they moved their heads. When Ronda came to class the next week, she told the group how enthusiastic she had been about this idea from the moment she heard it. In the following days, she was vividly aware of her neck being part of her whole spine as she moved. She was now experiencing remarkable improvement not only in her ability to do her yoga exercises, but also in all her daily movements. She reported feeling lighter and freer. She was astounded at the transformation that this new awareness of herself brought about.

Morty, a man in his late thirties, joined one of my long-term trainings. Soon it became clear to me, as well as the rest of the group, that Morty, a teacher and highly intellectual person, had the habit of being extremely critical. He was so critical, in fact, that he seemed mean. Yet it was obvious to me that Morty had very little knowledge of his habitual way of communicating and the negative effect it had on others. His awareness in this area of his life appeared to be almost nonexistent. His critical attitude seemed to prevent him from experiencing the joy and freedom that the rest of the class was enjoying. I expected him to drop out of the training, and yet he kept coming back. One day, during class, when he expressed yet another opinion in a critical and mean fashion, I decided to inform Morty about the impact he had on me. I told him that his critical way of communicating made it difficult for me to respond to him. I suggested that he become more aware of how he communicated, reminding him that he could experiment with new variations. He might slow down and look for kinder, more mindful and subtler ways of speaking. Morty was clearly stunned. He had no idea how his behavior affected others! A couple of days later, Morty raised his hand to ask a question in class. The room grew totally silent. Morty's tone of voice and the way he structured his question were caring and thoughtful, yet still communicated his point. What an amazing transformation! That initial awareness snowballed into remarkable changes in Morty's life. He has since moved to another town, made new friends, and has become much happier. His whole being gives out a sense of vitality and interest in life that I had never seen in him before.

Awareness gets us to apply our brain at its highest levels, giving us the power to make discoveries and create what otherwise would not be available to us. When lacking awareness, it is as if we are not present in our own lives. Without awareness, we are unable to truly be in the here and now, have little say in how our lives unfold, thus never quite living fully. The moment we become aware, it is as if the universe feeds us with new ideas, feelings, insights, and actions that lead us to remarkable transformations. Our brains are able to access their highest capacities, hence the transformations. Awareness is the most powerful tool we have as humans for reaching our greatest potential and therefore our greatest vitality.

EXERCISE 1   BE SAVVY, BE AWARE

Think of a situation in which you have noticed that you often have the same behaviors and experiences, ones that you don't like and wish to change. It could be a seemingly small matter, such as feeling irritated when finding that your partner has once again left the cap off the toothpaste. It might be the tension you feel in your shoulders when working at the computer. Or it could be what you experience when you discuss politics or social issues with a friend. The next time that situation comes up, slow down, pay attention, and become aware of some of your thoughts, feelings, and physical movements and of the reactions and feelings of the people around you. Notice that as you become increasingly aware, an opening is created for you to say, feel, think, or do something differently. Often, this is something you couldn't have anticipated ahead of time, something that works better for you than whatever you were doing before. Continue to bring your awareness to the same situation whenever it comes up until your experience is transformed and you are no longer a slave to your automatic responses and can experience the sense of freedom and empowerment that comes with it.

The Observer—the Heart of Awareness

Awareness requires the capacity for the observation of self and others. It is like shining a light that reveals something we had not seen before, changing not only our understanding of that thing, but often transforming the observer himself as well. Scientists who study awareness recognize the great challenge not only of researching it, but also of forming a precise definition of what awareness is. As with so many other subjects of scientific inquiry, they also know that while it may be difficult to define awareness, they can nevertheless observe it in action.

In my years of working with clients, I have witnessed over and over again the remarkable power of awareness. When I teach a movement lesson to a group, without failure there are great variations in the way the different participants execute the movement instructions I give them. When doing these movements in the way intended, a person will experience ease and pleasure. Some people will get the movement quickly and experience this ease and harmony immediately. Others will have their own variations and will experience some difficulty when they try to do the movement. From time to time, I will demonstrate with a participant who is having trouble with the movement so that everyone can see how these individual variations work—or don't work, as the case may be. I have the participant demonstrate her version of the movement to the rest of the group. It is obvious that all the participants are paying close attention to their bodies and sensations as they are moving, but that alone does not mean they are aware of what they are doing at that moment. After the chosen participant repeats that movement three or four times, I start pointing out some of the unique ways she is doing the movement. As I do this, she becomes aware of herself in a new way. Without exception, at this moment, the movement changes. Her previous way of moving shifts, and the way she moves becomes easier and smoother, with many of her previous limitations disappearing on the spot.

When I then ask this same person to go back to doing the movement in the way she did previously, she usually can't do it. She cannot repeat it because she was previously moving without awareness of what she was doing. I then describe to her what she previously did, talking her through her own original way of doing the movement so that she can re-create it. At that time, she becomes aware of the two different ways of moving, and as a result she begins to have a choice in what she does.

The awareness that results from demonstrating in this way, and which occurs whenever we *aware* in this way, is made possible because of our innate ability to step into being an observer. When we do so, it is as if we stand outside ourselves and witness what we are thinking, feeling, or doing. You may have experienced this for yourself, feeling like you were watching a movie in which you were an actor. *Merriam-Webster's Collegiate Dictionary* defines an observer as "a representative sent to observe but not participate officially in an activity." When we are observing, our task is to be aware, not to rush to action. Observing leads us to awareness. The human brain has remarkable observational capacities, and the more we use them on a regular basis, the more awareness we can bring to our lives.

There is extraordinary power in our observational abilities. Observing a thought, action, or feeling in ourselves creates new levels of organization and information in our brains. This not only allows the brain to create something new, but also prompts it to do so, and the end result is often transformational. Once awareness is brought to our thoughts, feelings, or actions in this way, it is impossible to go back to being unaware of that same thought, feeling, or action.

Awareness Is an Action

The role of awareness in our lives becomes clearer when we start thinking about it as an action. It is not a "thing," not something that we have or not, the same way we don't have "walking" or "talking." Awareness, like movement, is something that we do— or not. Just as I might say I am cooking, I am walking, I am dancing, I am thinking, or I am feeling, I propose that we learn to say I am *awaring*. If we are to more fully understand and benefit from the enormous potential of awareness, we need to start thinking of awareness as an active verb. This requires clear intentionality. It is a choice that we make. It is as far from automatic as you will ever get.

When we are *awaring*, we are drawing upon the full faculties of our amazing brains. We know that awaring emerges from the sheer complexity, that is, the enormous repertoire of possibilities our brains are able to make available to us. You experience awareness each time you look in the mirror and recognize the person staring back at you as you. You experience it every time you ruminate about an experience that you perhaps wish had had a different outcome. You experience it when you observe yourself in action and realize you could be doing it differently, more to your liking. You experience it when you become aware of habitual tendencies in someone else. You experience it when you become self-critical or when you take genuine pride in something you have accomplished. You experience it any time you set about improving the way you do something. You experience it every time you observe that your thoughts, feelings, and actions have an impact on others, with results that can either benefit or harm yourself, others, or the world around you.

Like any other skill, awareness requires practice. The more we bring the observer self into our lives, the better we get not only at awaring, but also at what it is we are doing. We benefit from the power of awareness to catapult our brains to higher and more-potent capacities of organization and creation. By awaring our movement, thoughts, feelings, and actions, we transform in ways that often seem miraculous. We can also apply our awaring skills in our relationships with others, with enlivening outcomes for them and ourselves.

EXERCISE 2   THE POWER OF AWARENESS

While spending many years in school sitting at desks writing and hours at our computers, plus being subjected to the general stresses of life, most of us experience tightness in our shoulders at one time or another. By the time we're in our thirties or forties, most of us can't freely lift our arms up to the sky, the way children do when they are excited, happy, and full of life. I invite you to do the following exercise and make sure to aware as you perform the movement. Become an active observer seeking to know what it is that you are feeling, thinking, and doing as you pay attention to your movements. Experience breaking through limitations and re-gaining the ability to do this movement that is so closely associated with feeling uplifted and alive.

PREPARATION

Wear comfortable, loose-fitting clothes. Have a straight-backed chair of a height that allows your thighs to be parallel to the floor and for you to have both feet flat on the floor. If necessary, place a book or two under your feet; if you have long legs, place a pillow under your pelvis so that your knees are at the same level as your hips.

THE EXERCISE

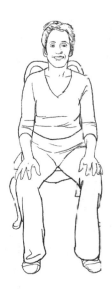

1. Sit at the edge of your chair, buttocks well supported, feet flat on the floor, at least a foot apart, with knees spread at about the same distance. Rest your hands palms down on the tops of your thighs. This is your neutral position for this lesson.

Take a moment to pay attention to your right shoulder, then your left one. Do they feel relaxed? Feel how far your right shoulder is from your right ear and your left shoulder from your left ear.

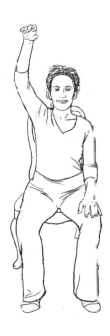

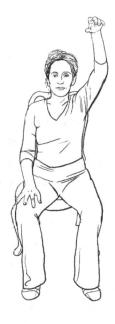

2. Still sitting at the edge of the chair, lift your right arm up toward the ceiling without forcing it. Aware what it feels like and how far you can lift your arm easily, without strain or pain, so that you can later evaluate and compare changes that have been created by this exercise. Put down your right arm and rest your hand on your thigh, as before. Now lift your left arm and aware how far you can comfortably lift it.

3. Continue sitting at the edge of the chair. Now gently and slowly begin moving your left shoulder forward and bring it back to place. Do not move your left arm or elbow forward, just your shoulder. Do this movement gently, without forcing, four or five times and stop. Be awaring of any movement elsewhere in your body as you move your shoulder forward.

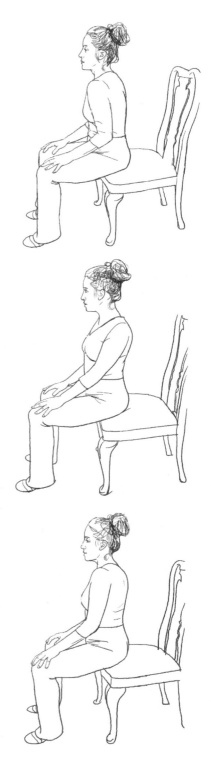

4. Now move that same left shoulder backward, very gently and slowly, and then come back to your neutral position four or five times—remembering to be awaring the whole time.

5. Still sitting at the edge of the chair, shift your weight slightly to the right buttock and slide your left hip forward and back. Note as you do this that your feet stay in place each time you move your left hip forward. Your left knee moves forward as your left hip and buttock move, and you arch your lower back on that side. Do this movement four or five times, gently. Rest for a moment. Feel the contact of your right buttock with the chair and compare it to the left.

6. Now shift your weight to your right buttock again and move your left hip backward, then return to neutral, four or five times. Be awaring of what happens throughout your back and spine as you do this movement. Rest for a moment.

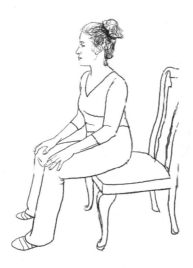

7. This time, simultaneously move your left shoulder and left hip forward and then move them at the same time backward. Be awaring of your whole body. Do this movement four or five times. Rest for a moment.

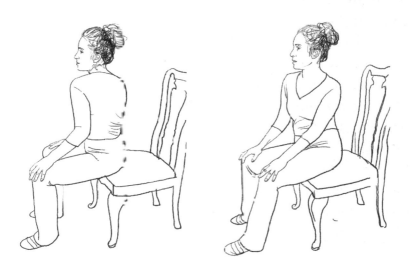

8. Sitting at the edge of your chair, move your left shoulder and left hip in opposite directions. When you move the left shoulder forward, move your left hip backward, and vice versa. Here you need to be awaring to make sure that you are doing what you think you are doing. Repeat this whole movement three or four times. Rest for a moment.

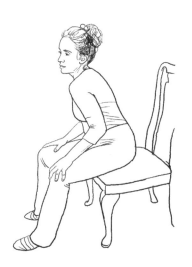 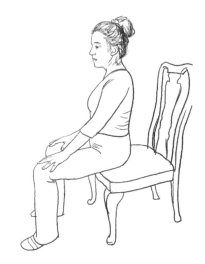

9. Now simply sit at the edge of the chair and be aware of how your left shoulder feels; is it lower than when you started this exercise? It is more relaxed? Compare your left and right shoulders. Lift your left arm up toward the ceiling; does it feel different? Does it lift higher? Better? Easier? Now lift your right arm toward the ceiling; you might feel how different it is compared with your left arm.

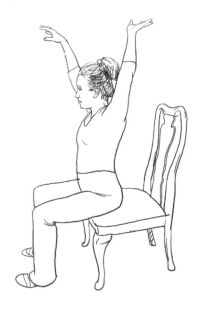

AWARING IN EVERYDAY LIFE

My friend Barry was leaving his Las Vegas hotel after a very busy three-day conference. He was tired, somewhat irritable, and anxious to get to the airport as quickly as possible. As he went out to the curb, he found there were throngs of people waiting for cabs at three valet lines. Barry noticed that one line was moving faster than others, and there seemed to be a good deal of excitement at the head of it, with eruptions of laughter from time to time. Curious, and wanting to get a cab as fast as possible, he joined that line.

As Barry got closer to the front of the line, he saw that this valet had a big smile on his face, was talking a lot, and was very animated. He appeared to have incredible rapport with the people and to be entertaining them as they waited.

When Barry got even closer, he observed that people were handing this valet $10 and $20 tips as he was helping them into their cabs. Barry's immediate thought was "There's no way in the world I'm going to give this guy twenty bucks!" He watched carefully as the valet helped an older couple into their cab.

"I hope you had a great trip, sir, and that you and your daughter here had a wonderful time," the valet said.

Both the husband and the wife laughed as he said this. While Barry had heard other valets use a similar line, there was something different about how this valet did it. He wasn't just being automatic, following a rote script; instead, he seemed to notice and be aware of something unique in each of his customers. His awaring extended beyond himself to others. He was right there in the present with each one, ready to serve them and elevate their experience.

When two young and somewhat timid college students came to the head of the line, the valet grinned from ear to ear and asked them, "Did you have a great time in Vegas?" When they nodded and smiled shyly, he said, "Yeah, yeah! That's great. And I want you to know that what happens in Vegas stays in Vegas." They giggled, as if sharing a secret with him, and he nodded to acknowledge what they were feeling. My friend, still skeptical, began to recognize what was different about this valet: He seemed to be aware enough of each customer to be able to say just the right thing, a few words that fit them uniquely well. In that brief encounter, the valet sent each person on the way feeling a little happier.

As Barry was approaching the head of the line, he was eagerly anticipating his turn, wondering what this guy could possibly say to him that might cause him to shell out a $20 tip. Then he was next in line. The valet hailed a cab, turned to my friend, bowed, and exclaimed, "Oh my God, I finally get to meet Brad Pitt!" My friend, who does somewhat resemble Brad Pitt, and who pays particular attention to his appearance, couldn't help but feel good. He laughed and handed the valet a $20 bill as he climbed into his cab.

My friend told me, "I know I'm no Brad Pitt, but I sure felt good for a few hours, and every time I think about this incident, I feel good about myself once again."

Another friend of mine shared the story of a garbage collector in the neighborhood where she lived. He was no ordinary garbage collector. When someone forgot to put his disposal can out at the curb, this guy did something quite out of the ordinary. He took the time to go and get it, if at all possible. He noticed when there was garbage or debris on the ground and was always quick to pick it up. He was cheerful and outgoing, never failing to say hello or giving a wave as he passed. It was obvious that he took a high level of interest in his work. He was not only attentive to details, noticing things that seemed invisible to others, but he used these observations to aware and take actions that elevated his and his customers' experience. He took actions other garbage collectors didn't take. Gradually, the people on his route noticed what he was doing and recognized how his efforts contributed to their community. Their admiration for him grew.

This man inspired the community to such an extent that when

it was learned that one of his children had a serious illness, requiring hospitalization, the people got together and raised a few thousand dollars to help out with medical expenses.

In both cases, there is tremendous vitality in what these men are doing. Here they are, doing work that many people would find boring and even beneath their dignity, but by awaring as they are doing their jobs, they are elevating what they do, themselves, and those around them. By bringing lots of awaring to their activities, they draw upon infinite numbers of observations and nuances, and as a result engage in their lives in ways that are vital, innovative, and personally satisfying at the end of the day.

Jacob Bronowski, the author of the popular book and creator of the public television series *The Ascent of Man,* speaks well to this point. He said, "The most powerful drive in the ascent of man is his pleasure in his own skill. He loves to do what he does well and, having done it well, he loves to do it better." And awaring is essential for that to happen.

We all possess this capacity we call awareness, by which we are able to observe, know, and change ourselves. But first and foremost we need to *choose awaring*. When we follow our automatic patterns and habits, very little is required of us, except the expenditure of energy. Over time, that way of living our lives can leave us feeling stifled, stuck, and even hopeless. If we wish to live our lives with vitality, we no longer have the laissez-faire luxury of falling back on prewired and preprogrammed ways of operating in the world. Awareness is a source of freedom. When observing ourselves and infusing our lives with awareness, there are greater and greater openings, opportunities for creating something new, something different, something better.

The more we use the skill of awaring, the more it expands, becoming stronger and more integral with the inner workings of our brains. Our lives become richer, more varied, and we are no longer automatons treading the same paths day after day. Instead, we follow our true human path. We bring more to life, and life in return rewards us with the vitality we are seeking.

EXERCISE 3 AWARENESS

WHAT'S YOUR VITALITY QUOTIENT?

On a scale of 1 to 5, rate yourself in each of the following statements, with 5 being always, 3 being occasionally, 1 being never.

1. I recognize the value of awareness of self and others.

2. I am mindful of how awareness impacts the quality of my life.

3. I am inspired by people who exhibit high levels of awareness.

4. When I encounter a problem, I seek to become aware of what is happening within me and around me.

5. I am aware of the impact my words and tone of voice have on others.

6. I quickly become aware whenever I move in ways that strain my body, and experiment with new ways of moving.

7. I seek to recognize when I sound or act like an automaton and immediately begin awaring.

Score Yourself
24–35 points = high
15–23 points = medium
1–14 points = low

Go through the seven statements above and choose the ones on which you scored the lowest. Take some time to think about ways to improve your scores in those areas. The statements themselves will guide you.

Move into Life

*There is nothing in a caterpillar that tells you it's going
to be a butterfly.*

—BUCKMINSTER FULLER

Vitality is within your grasp no matter what your age or life
circumstances. As we've seen, reduced vitality is not the result of
stress, lifestyle, injury, illness, or aging per se. It is the result of habits,
beliefs, and limitations—some that we're conscious of, some we're not
—that can be changed. With NeuroMovement and the Nine Essentials
as guidelines—*Moving with Attention, the Learning Switch, Subtlety,
Variation, Slow, Flexible Goals, Enthusiasm, Imagination and
Dreams,* and *Awareness*— we can provide our brains with what they
require for creating high levels of vitality easily and quickly.

By incorporating the Essentials in your everyday life, you create
the conditions for your brain to make use of the stimulation
coming from both inside and outside your self, turning it into new,
more refined information that improves the quality and ease of
what you do, how you think and feel, and how you experience
your life. Thanks to the wisdom and practices of the Nine Essentials, you are no longer limited to relying solely on what
you already know; instead, you will move more powerfully into life

with increased flexibility and creativity, filled with the delight of discovering new possibilities. Like a healthy young child, you will become increasingly aware of the richness, variety, and diversity that is all around you.

By now, you may have noticed that at the heart of the Anat Baniel Method, NeuroMovement, and the Nine Essentials is a process called *differentiation*. Differentiation is the process by which cells change and come to differ from one another in order to perform specialized functions. Differentiation in the brain involves the formation and organization of *neurons* (brain cells) and *synapses* (connections between the cells) that form precise nerve circuits (patterns)--whole constellations of neurons creating unique functions. Differentiation is a fundamental process of life; it is the development from the one to the many, from the simple to the complex, and from the same to the unique.

Scientists are able to measure and track the process of differentiation as it is taking place in the brain. They are able to show that as we gain a new skill, or improve on an existing one, more brain cells get involved—the brain map associated with that skill gets larger. But that is not all. At the same time, each brain cell is responsible for a smaller part, which allows for finer control. So if you are learning, let's say, how to play the piano, your refined movements develop because more brain cells and more synapses (brain connections) become associated with the movements of your fingers, and as you get better at playing, each cell serves a smaller and smaller part of your hand. As a result, you move your hand in a more precise, complex, and refined way. That refinement of movement in your fingers is differentiation in action. While differentiation is most active in the first few years following birth, the Nine Essentials reawaken differentiation in the brain and make vitality a constant in our lives.

So often the arc of life looks like a bell-shaped curve. Vitality and differentiation rise quickly in the first part of life, plateaus for a while at the top of the bell, and then starts going down, sometimes precipitously. The downturn may feel inevitable, but by building our natural capacities for differentiation, we can have a brain that continues to form new connections, and create new patterns at a tremendous rate, filling all our years with the boundless energy, optimism, constant change, and wonder of our early years.

More Than Just the Sum of the Parts

There's a Hebrew word, *shichlul,* that describes the role the Nine Essentials play in upgrading our brains and enhancing our vitality. It is roughly translated as "improvement and refinement through increased complexity." This does not mean that our lives become more complicated or difficult as we refine and improve. On the contrary, as *shichlul* takes place, in this case through the Nine Essentials, the experience of our lives is one of greater simplicity, ease, and pleasure. Shichlul *makes the impossible possible, the possible comfortable, and the comfortable elegant.*

When I am teaching in seminars the relationship between vitality and increased differentiation and complexity, I often draw the outline of a duck on a whiteboard. Then I draw four or five rather large, random shapes of simple puzzle pieces. I ask my students to put those pieces together so that they match the image of the duck. They quickly note, of course, that it can't be done. No matter how they put those pieces together, they're still not going to make a duck. The pieces are too big and none of the shapes quite match the curves of the duck.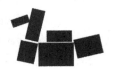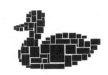

I then start drawing lots of very tiny shapes on the board: triangles, circles, squares, amorphous shapes, and even simple dots. I ask the students to imagine taking as many of these shapes as they need and creating the picture of a duck with them. Everyone quickly realizes that this would be easy; you simply use these tiny pieces to fill the space defined by the outline of the duck. In fact, with the same tiny pieces, you could also create the image of a mouse, a car, a cat, a human being, or an entire landscape.

This, I tell them, is a graphic example of differentiation and the richness of possibility that differentiation affords us. Imagine that you had in your brain only four or five big puzzle pieces. With only a few chunky resources like this, your brain would be severely limited; your experience of life would be narrowed down to a very small range of possibilities. In fact, it would not take long before every hour and every day of your life began to look pretty much like every other. You would often feel stuck. There would be many mishaps. You'd feel frustrated with your life and with your lack of skills. You'd tend to feel like the world was out of control and that you were a victim of your life rather than being at the helm. With the extreme limitation of resources, your brain would have a difficult time making much sense of the outside world at all. You would feel drained of energy and vitality.

If life becomes dull, frustrating, and seemingly out of control with such limited resources, what's the opposite side of that equation? How would our lives be changed when we have access to volumes and volumes of more and more refined resources? Do the math, and you begin to see that our possibilities, and thus our choices and our freedom to act effectively and powerfully, would grow extremely fast. If I use all of the elements that I have at any given time and just change their order around, when I have only one piece—A—there is only one possible combination I can do with that resource. If I have two pieces—A and B—there are two possibilities: AB and BA. Add one more resource and the fun begins: $1 \times 2 \times 3 = 6$ possibilities; add one more and you have $1 \times 2 \times 3 \times 4 = 24$; add one more and you have $1 \times 2 \times 3 \times 4 \times 5 = 120$ possibilities; at six, you have 720 possibilities, and at seven, you have 5,040 possibilities. By adding only nine more resources to your original one, you will end up with 3,628,800 options! If, on top of that, I can combine any number of those elements, not just all of them all the time, and place them in changing orders, then the number of possibilities grows even faster. And that is what the Nine Essentials are all about. They give your brain what it needs to transform you, to create solutions you couldn't have known to ask for. Small changes create large numbers of possibilities, and the greater the number of possibilities that your brain has at the ready, the more freedom you have to live life fully and authentically.

In a very real way, the Nine Essentials provide our brains with what they need to reinvent themselves—and thus our vitality—over and over again, always moving toward freer, more creative and effective ways of doing and being. We keep progressing and evolving, becoming more and more who we were born to be. In the spiritual traditions of the Israeli people, *shichlul* was the way to attaining the highest levels of personal achievement and spiritual fulfillment—what was often referred to as the *crowning beauty.*

Think of world-class violin player Itzhak Perlman, a musician who is the very essence of vitality. At concerts, he seems to be having a wonderful time. The music flowing from his violin is exquisite, moving us, charming us, and transporting us into a place that is at times ecstatic. Perlman makes it look so easy, and the music so beautiful that we are seduced into believing that we must surely be feeling what he is feeling; he has made it possible for us to experience at least some of what he is feeling. This is the very essence of *shichlul,* for his brain is providing ongoing and infinitely complex organization of movement—constant invention and improvement, refinement, and complexity—drawn from years of playing the violin and never stopping to do his own version of the Nine Essentials.

Does this mean that we all have to become Itzhak Perlmans to have the vitality we are seeking? Not at all. It is not in *what* the profession or activity is that our vitality lies, but in the *how* we go about doing it.

Research shows that hours of solving crossword puzzles, travel-ing to new places, or doing rote exercises do not necessarily in-crease differentiation, nor do they by themselves promote the creation of new connections in the brain; thus, these are not, in and of themselves, sure ways for increasing vitality. On the other hand, if approached with the guidance of the Nine Essentials, even the most mundane and seemingly automatic activities can immediately begin increasing complexity and refinement, triggering *shichlul*.

Two of my students, Matthew, a car mechanic and an owner of a car-repair shop, and his wife, Karen, a massage therapist, de-cided to leave their work behind and take a vacation. They rented a small summer cottage on the beach for a few weeks. Upon ar-rival, they discovered that the cottage did not have a dishwasher. First they felt a bit upset, being so accustomed to having a dish-washer at home. After a short discussion, they decided they would take turns washing dishes. When Matthew's turn came, Karen, who was in the other room, heard lots of commotion and banging sounds. When she went into the kitchen, she found Matthew fran-tically rushing through the task. Later, she noticed that some of the washed dishes still had food remnants on them and a couple were chipped. Matthew, on the other hand, didn't seem to notice anything.

After a few days of this, Karen decided to bring the subject up with Matthew. She gently drew his attention to what she had ob-served. Matthew was at first surprised and a bit defensive. But soon he became curious. As a car mechanic, he surely knew how to use his hands very well. Being aware of the Nine Essentials, he realized what he'd been doing; instead of approaching washing the dishes as something new, he had been doing it automatically, the way he normally loaded the dishwasher. He decided that the next time it was his turn to wash the dishes, he would apply some of the Nine Essentials. He became enthusiastic about the opportunity to experiment with washing the dishes. He moved more slowly as he was doing the task and brought close attention to his movements. He experimented with different ways of piling up the washed dishes to dry. He became aware of how much excess force he was using in his hands and arms. Once he reduced the force, he became much more coordinated and was able to feel and notice when the dishes were clean. As he approached the new task in this way, he actually began to enjoy the experience itself, the sensations of warmth and the feeling of the sudsy water, the focus of his attention as he worked, and, afterward, a sense of focus that he came away with. He even told Karen about what he was experiencing and said how he no longer viewed washing the dishes as something to finish as quickly as possible, but as an extension of his vacation.

The rest of the summer, Matthew continued to experiment with improving his system of washing the dishes. When Matthew returned to work, to his amazement, he discovered that both his skill and his enjoyment as a car mechanic had been upgraded to a whole new level. His old excitement at fixing cars, which he hadn't felt for a long time, had returned. The refinement he developed in relation to washing dishes transferred to other areas of his life. When he saw me in the fall, he excitedly told me the story and said, "This stuff is for real! The Essentials really work. And who would have ever thought that learning to wash dishes would carry over into my job?"

THE NINE ESSENTIALS: A SHORT REVIEW

Each and every time I work with people in my practice or workshops, I'm astounded by the immediacy and scope of the changes that occur through the application of the Nine Essentials. I am reminded, over and over again, of how, when we take an already remarkable brain that is highly complex and developed and propel it to come back to life, it will grow and reorganize itself. Each time we do this, the miraculous just keeps happening.

I encourage you to begin experimenting with the Nine Essentials. You can follow them in order, as presented in this book. You can select the ones to which you are most strongly attracted. Or you can choose to start with the ones for which you have found you have the lowest quotient score. At first, it is best to focus on one Essential at a time. Do that for a day, or a few days. You may first try the exercises described in the chapter about the Essential you are working on. Then look for opportunities to introduce that Essential into as many areas in your daily life as you can. Then move to the next Essential. After you have worked with all of the Nine Essentials, you can apply them in your everyday life a few at a time. Whenever you want to increase your vitality, or get past being stuck, feeling limited, feeling bored, or being in pain, in any area of your life, begin introducing the Nine Essentials to that area.

You may have already discovered that the principles and methods described in these pages can be applied in a variety of ways, so always feel free to apply the Nine Essentials in any way that appeals to you. Remember, there is no way for you to go wrong while evolving and growing; there is only your way, a way that is teeming with new information and possibilities.

* **MOVEMENT WITH ATTENTION.** Movement is everywhere. You can choose any movement you are already doing in your life and bring attention to it. You can also bring new and more movement into your life. Remember that movement involves your body, your thoughts, your feelings, and your emotions.

* **TURNING ON THE LEARNING SWITCH.** Learning is life. Without learning, we would never be able to do anything. Rather than being prewired or preprogrammed at birth, we are wired to learn, and to develop our human capacities. As the years pass, we tend to rely on what we already know. We act automatically and stop dancing with life, in the now, in a powerful and vibrant way. When you turn on your learning switch, you turn on your life.

* **SUBTLETY.** Reducing the force (subtlety) increases your sensitivity and allows your brain to turn stimulation into new information.

- **VARIATIONS.** Provide your brain with the richness of information it needs to create a greater variety of possibilities in your feelings, thoughts, and actions. Variations help increase your awareness and lift you out of rigidity and stuckness.

- **SLOW.** Slowing down wakes up your brain's attention and increases your ability to notice what is going on and create the new. Remember, by going fast, you can only do what you already know.

- **ENTHUSIASM.** Enthusiasm tells your brain what is important to you, amplifies it, making it stand out, and infuses it with energy to grow more. Enthusiasm is a powerful energy that lifts and inspires you and others.

- **HOLDING GOALS LOOSELY.** Freeing yourself from the compulsion to achieve goals a certain way at a certain time makes room for new possibilities to form, leading you to successfully accomplish what is important to you.

- **IMAGINING AND DREAMING.** Your imagination and dreams give you the ability to create something that has never been there before, transcending your current limitations and leading you to develop your authentic life path.

- **AWARENESS.** *Awaring*—knowing, and knowing that you know—is the opposite of automaticity and compulsion. It is a unique human capacity that can catapult us to remarkable heights.

N THE IMAGE OF GOD

In every religious and spiritual tradition, we find the concept that man and woman are born in the image of God, or perhaps a higher order known by other names. Some say the truth of this cannot be proven scientifically. And yet, as I think of the thousands of miracles I've witnessed over the more than thirty years in my work, it is the creative capacities of the human brain, and the endless inventiveness of human expression, that I feel most reflect this truth. We were created to create, for it is through our creative capacity that we humans are able to grow and expand our skills and awareness, evolve in our personal development, and experience the full delight, energy, and vitality we are capable of achieving.

Somehow in the attributes we share with the Divine, there is an implied responsibility to make use of what we have been given and to seek whatever it takes to make life a little better, richer, and more vibrant each day. There is a direction to human life, a curve we can create, always moving from chaos and emptiness to greater order and richness. There is no perfection toward which we must aspire, no fixed standards of the right or correct way to do things in order to have vitality, success, and satisfaction. Rather, our challenge is to be involved in the process of continued exploration. When we aren't, when we stop for too long, we begin experiencing the stuckness, the fatigue, the waning of interest, the defeat—the loss of vitality.

Right now, in this instant, your brain is at the ready to resume its job of figuring out new, more evolved and satisfying ways for you to act and be. It is my conviction that the Anat Baniel Method NeuroMovement and the Nine Essentials, will always serve you in your pursuit of those intentions.

The miraculous occurs whenever we start applying the skills and knowledge I describe in this book, since these provide our brains with exactly what they need to thrive. While we can't peek inside our brains and see their inner workings, we can experience what they do in the ways our bodies feel, in the effortlessness or grace of our movements, in the increased clarity of our thoughts, in the feelings of joy and optimism and accomplishment. This is what we all long for, that sense of freedom, the feeling of personal power, of ever-growing mastery—of vitality.

Think of yourself as a great work of art in progress, as a miracle or, more accurately, infinite miracles that have already occurred and will continue to occur throughout your years. Dance with the present. Meet each moment with curiosity, wonder, and aliveness! With NeuroMovement and the Nine Essentials of the Anat Baniel Method, I know you will achieve lifelong vitality.

Notes

VITALITY AND YOUTHFULNESS

7   **1.8 million connections per second:** L. Eliot, 1999, *What's Going on in There? How the Brain and Mind Develop in the First Five Years of Life* (New York: Bantam), 27.

8   **Our brains thrive when creating new information:** Neurobiologists have known that a novel environment sparks exploration and learning, but, until recently, very little was known about whether the brain really prefers novelty as such. Now, researchers Nico Bunzeck and Emrah Duzel report studies with humans showing that the major "novelty center" of the brain—called the substantia nigra/ventral tegmental area (SN/VTA)—does respond to novelty as such, and this novelty motivates the brain to explore, seeking a reward. Bunzeck and Duzel found that novelty enhanced learning in the subjects. N. Bunzeck and E. Duzel, 2006, "Absolute Coding of Stimulus Novelty in the Human Substantia Nigra/VTA." *Neuron* 51 (Aug. 3):369–379; Reported in "Pure Novelty Spurs the Brain," *Medical News Today*, August 6, 2006.

15   **We have only to provide our brains with new information:** Nobel laureate Gerald M. Edelman states that "the brains of higher level animals autonomously construct patterned responses to environments that are full of novelty." G. M. Edelman, 2005, *Wider Than the Sky* (New Haven, Conn.: Yale University Press), 38–39.

17   **Until quite recently, it was believed:** S. Begley, 2007, "How the Brain Rewires Itself," *Time*, January 19. It was only in 1999 that Torsten Wiesel, who won the Nobel Prize with David Hubel in 1981 for his studies of the development of the visual cortex, after

much public denial, admitted in print that adult neuroplasticity was a genuine phenomenon. T. N. Wiesel, 1999, "Early Explorations of the Development and Plasticity of the Visual Cortex: A Personal View," *Journal of Neurobiology* 41(1):7–9.

17   science has now shown that *neurogenesis:* Animal studies over the last decade have overturned the assumption that the adult brain is "fixed," showing that *neurogenesis*—the formation of new nerve cells—can be induced easily with exercise in some parts of the brain. A recent study published in the *Proceedings of the National Academy of Sciences* extended that principle to humans for the first time. After working out for three months, all the subjects appeared to sprout new neurons. With moderate athletic activity, or regular daily exercise, our muscles release a variety of chemicals that enter the brain and trigger the production of certain neurotransmitters that fuel activities associated with higher thinking. New brain cells start branching out, sprouting new neurons and establishing new connections with other groups of brain cells. A. C. Pereira, D. E. Huddleston, A. M. Brickman, A. A. Sosunov, R. Hen, G. M. McKhann, R. Sloan, F. H. Gage, T. R. Brown, and S. A. Small, 2007, "An in Vivo Correlate of Exercise-Induced Neurogenesis in the Adult Dentate Gyrus," *Proceedings of the National Academy of Sciences* 104(13):5638–5643. Reported in M. Carmichael, 2007, "Stronger, Faster, Smarter: Exercise Does More Than Build Muscles and Help Prevent Heart Disease; New Science Shows That It Also Boosts Brainpower—and May Offer Hope in the Battle Against Alzheimer's," *Newsweek,* March 26.

17   In recent research by neuroscientist Alvaro Pascual-Leone: See chapter 9.

18   Our brains are organized through movement: See chapter 2.

18   combined with attention: "In all three of the cortical systems where scientists have documented neuroplasticity—the primary auditory cortex, somatosensory cortex, and motor cortex—the variable determining whether or not the brain changes is . . . the attentional state of the animal." J. Schwartz and S. Begley, 2003, *The Mind and the Brain: Neuroplasticity and the Power of Mental Force* (New York: ReganBooks), 338.

One. Movement with Attention—Wake Up to Life

23   **our simplest thoughts and feelings involve movement:** It has long been known that a nerve impulse is conducted along nerve fibers by the movement of charged ions across the cell membrane and then the movement of neurotransmitter from one cell to the next at the junctions between cells, but it has only recently been discovered just how much movement is involved in the actual structure of the nerve terminals. "Now, after peering closer than ever before at the elaborate branches of individual nerve cells, scientists have discovered that the twigs, known as dendrites, are decorated with tiny ornaments, called dendritic spines—and that the ornaments can move." Carl T. Hall, 1999, "Structures in Motion Seen at Synapses—Discovery Could Revamp View of Brain Function," *San Francisco Chronicle,* January 5. See E. R. Kandel, 2006, *In Search of Memory: The Emergence of a New Science of Mind.* (New York: W. W. Norton); A. Matus, 2000, "Actin-Based Plasticity in Dendritic Spines," *Science* 290:754–758.

24   **Within your brain are billions of brain cells:** At birth, the brain contains something in the region of 100 billion neurons, each of which connects to anywhere between a few thousand to one hundred thousand other neurons through specialized junctions called synapses. A conservative estimate of the total number of synapses in the adult brain is 100 trillion. The formation of synapses begins in the cerebral cortex, for example, during the seventh week of gestation and continues well into childhood. It is estimated that at its peak, each neuron forms an average of fifteen thousand connections. This equates to a rate of formation of 1.8 million synapses per second during the period from the second month in utero until the child's second birthday. Not all of these synapses survive. See A. Gopnik, A. N. Meltzoff, and P. K. Kuhl, 1999, *The Scientist in the Crib: Minds, Brains and How Children Learn* (New York: William Morrow), 181–186; L. Eliot, 1999, *What's Going On in There? How the Brain and Mind Develop in the First Five Years of Life* (New York: Bantam) 27–32; and J. J. Ratey, 2000, *A User's Guide to the Brain* (New York: Pantheon), 26.

25   **Movement is the language of your brain:** Nobel laureate Gerald M. Edelman states, "The brain's motor functions . . . are . . . critically important, not just for the regulation of movement, but also for forming images and concepts." He says, "In the mammalian nervous system, perceptual categorization is carried out by

interactions between sensory and motor systems . . . [we first] sample the world of signals by movement and attention and then . . . categorize these signals as coherent through . . . synchronization of neuronal groups." G. M. Edelman, 2005, *Wider Than the Sky* (New Haven, Conn.: Yale University Press), 23, 49.

25   **through *bringing attention to our movements:*** One of the great pioneers of neuroplasticity research is Michael Merzenich of UCSF. For an excellent and approachable overview of his work, see N. Doidge, 2007, *The Brain That Changes Itself* (New York: Viking Penguin) especially chap. 3, "Redesigning the Brain," 45–92.

Merzenich has shown that a prerequisite for plastic change in the brain is attention. Initially, he demonstrated this by training owl monkeys in a sensory discrimination task, rewarding their success in paying attention to a stimulus to their hand with food. In a parallel experiment, he distracted their attention by rewarding attention to an auditory stimulus. Plastic changes were only present in the areas of the brain corresponding to the specific area of attention, that is, somatosensory or auditory. G. H. Recanzone, M. M. Merzenich, W. M. Jenkins, K. A. Grajski, and H. R. Dinse, 1992b, "Topographic Reorganization of the Hand Representation in Cortical Area 3b of Owl Monkeys Trained in a Frequency Discrimination Task," *Journal of Neurophysiology* 67:1031–1056.

In 1996, he and his colleagues demonstrated such plastic change in the motor cortex. The experiments trained squirrel monkeys to retrieve food pellets from four food wells of differing sizes. The results showed that plastic change occurred in the motor cortex and suggested that use-dependent plastic reorganization occurs in a number of associated structures, including the motor cortex, the basal ganglia, the cerebellum, and the spinal cord. R. J. Nudo, G. W. Milliken, W. M. Jenkins, and M. M. Merzenich, 1996, "Use-Dependent Alterations of Movement Representations in Primary Motor Cortex of Adult Squirrel Monkeys," *Journal of Neuroscience* 16(2):785–807.

30   **Movement coupled with attention . . . serve as a rich source of information to the brain:** Much of twentieth-century neuroscientific research centered on the study of cortical sensory perception, particularly vision. Much of that research was done in isolation from brain functioning as a whole. Alain Berthoz, director of the Laboratory of Physiology of Perception and Action at the Collège de France, elegantly presents perception as an action whose devel-

opment is critically dependent upon movement and the information that movement provides. See A. Berthoz, 2000, *The Brain's Sense of Movement*, trans. Giselle Weiss (Cambridge, Mass.: Harvard University Press).

35   **What is missing is attention:** To quote Merzenich, "Experience coupled with attention leads to physical changes in the structure and functioning of the nervous system." M. M. Merzenich and R. C. Decharms, "Neural Representations, Experience and Change," in *The Mind-Brain Continuum,* ed. R. Llinás and P. S. Churchland (Cambridge, MA: MIT Press, 1996), 77.

40   **In his book *The Power of Now:*** E. Tolle, 1999, *The Power of Now* (Novato, CA: New World Library) 97.

40   **you see brand-new clusters of cells lighting up:** A number of imaging studies have now shown this and publish the images; Dick Passingham of Oxford University used positron-emission tomography (PET) to study differences in brain activity between new learning and automatic performance in normal volunteers. Scans showed high levels of activity in the prefrontal cortex during new learning, but not once the performance became routine. By paying special attention to the now-automatic task, the prefrontal cortex became metabolically active once more. M. Jueptner, K. M. Stephan, C. D. Frith, D. J. Brooks, R. S. J. Frackowiak, and R. E. Passingham, 1997, "Anatomy of Motor Learning: I. Frontal Cortex and Attention to Action," *Journal of Neurophysiology* 77(3):1313–1324.

      Another study headed by Heidi Johansen-Berg, also of Oxford University, used functional magnetic resonance imagery (fMRI). It concluded that "robust . . . widespread attentional effects are found in multiple areas responsible for motor control." H. Johansen-Berg and P. M. Matthews, 2002. "Attention to Movement Modulates Activity in Sensori-Motor Areas, Including Primary Motor Cortex," *Experimental Brain Research* 142(1):13–24.

42   **excellent at creating set "templates" or "programs":** Gerald Edelman states that "the brains of higher-level animals autonomously construct patterned responses to environments that are full of novelty." Edelman, *Wider Than the Sky,* 38–39.

44   **specifically the brain's organizational abilities:** Esther Thelen and Linda Smith refer to Edelman when they propose that for babies "the correlated activity of looking and reaching [i.e., attention and movement] engenders real changes in brain circuits." E. Thelen and L. B. Smith, 1994, *A Dynamic Systems Approach to the*

Development of Cognition and Action (Cambridge, Mass.: MIT Press), 305.

44   **Our brains crave new information:** See chapter 1.

46   **"It ain't what you do . . .:** This was first recorded by Ella Fitzgerald in 1939 as "T'ain't what you do, it's the way that you do it." Louis Armstrong released it as "T'ain't what you do, it's the way cha do it."

Two. The Learning Switch—Bring in the New

48   **a process I call *turning on the learning switch:*** The switch is a metaphor, not an anatomical entity, describing the clearly observable shift of a person into a learning mode as akin to the change brought about by turning on a light in a darkened room. "We all know that such a state exists, we just don't know what the mechanism is." Mark Latash (author of *Neurophysiological Basis of Human Movement* [Champaign, Ill.: Human Kinetics, 1998]), Distinguished Professor of Kinesiology, Pennsylvania State University, in a conversation with the author.

The following paragraphs represent some views as to the measurable characteristics of such a state and its potential mechanisms.

1. Electrical activity of the brain can be measured as "brain waves" by an electroencephalogram on the surface of the skull. Certain patterns characteristic of childhood become less common in adulthood (e.g., so-called theta waves) but are seen in dreaming or "creative" states and meditation. Electrical and other mechanisms of alertness are discussed in B. Oken and M. Salinsky, 1992, "Alertness and Attention: Basic Science and Electrophysiologic Correlates," *Journal of Clinical Neurophysiology* 9(4):480–494.

2. The most common cells in the brain are not neurons (nerve cells) but glial cells. They support the nerve cells structurally, regulate the environment around synapses and are dramatically altered by challenging experiences and learning opportunities. They thus have the potential to maintain a chemical learning state in the brain. W. K. Dong and W. T. Greenough, 2004, "Plasticity of Nonneuronal Brain Tissue: Roles in Developmental Disorders," *Mental Retardation and Developmental Disabilities Research Reviews,* 10:85–90.

3. Nobel Prize winner Eric Kandel has done much research on the conversion of short-term to long-term memory. He has identified a self-propogating mechanism based on a short protein fragment called a prion. Prions had previously only been known to be

associated with devastating neurological diseases like BSE (mad cow disease). C. H. Bailey, E. R. Kandel, and K. Si, 2004, "The Persistence of Long-Term Memory: A Molecular Approach to Self-Sustaining Changes in Learning-Induced Synaptic Growth," *Neuron* 44(1):49–57; A. Barco, C. H. Bailey, and E. R. Kandel, 2006, "Common Molecular Mechanisms in Explicit and Implicit Memory," *Journal of Neurochememistry* 97(6):1520–1533. Kandel also talks of experiments in which he bred mice deficient in a particular gene whose learning in response to a stimulus was greatly enhanced. "As a result these mice were brilliant; they had a much stronger spatial memory than normal mice." E. R. Kandel, 2007 *In Search of Memory: The Emergence of a New Science of Mind* (New York: W. W. Norton), 293.

4. Michael Merzenich has done research on the role of a particular brain structure called the basal nucleus and its role in selecting behaviorally important stimuli and ignoring irrelevant ones. See note on pages 270–271.

49 a process that brain researchers call "pruning": See K. McAuliffe, 2007, "Life of the Brain—Midlife: Adult Behaviors," in "The Brain: An Owner's Manual," *Discover* (Spring): 13–14. McAuliffe quotes research by Jay McLelland, a psychologist from Stanford University. Japanese newborns, like all others, have the potential ability to perceive the difference between "r" and "l," but their language doesn't contain those distinct sounds. As they grow older, the patterns learned from their experience become more and more entrenched. As adults, Japanese speakers can no longer distinguish the two sounds. B. D. McCandliss, J. A. Fiez, A. Protopapas, M. Conway, and J. L. McClelland, 2002, "Success and Failure in Teaching the [r]-[l] Contrast to Japanese Adults: Predictions of a Hebbian Model of Plasticity and Stabilization in Spoken Language Perception," *Cognitive, Affective and Behavioral Neuroscience* 2:89–108. Such grooving as we age can be demonstrated as a reduction of gray matter on MRI scans. N. Raz, U. Lindenberger, K. M. Rodrigue, K. M. Kennedy, D. Head, A. Williamson, C. Dahle, D. Gerstorf, and J. D. Acker, 2005, "Regional Brain Changes in Aging Healthy Adults: General Trends, Individual Differences and Modifiers," *Cerebral Cortex* 15:1676–1689.

49 "cells that fire together, wire together": In a famous passage in his 1949 book *The Organization of Behaviour* (New York: Wiley), Hebb proposed a neural mechanism for learning: "When an axon of cell A is near enough to excite a cell B and repeatedly

or persistently takes part in firing it, some growth process or metabolic change takes place in one or both cells such that A's efficiency, as one of the cells firing B, is increased." In other words, the more often one nerve cell excites another, the more likely they are to fire together in the future, or "Cells that fire together wire together." The source of this latter version is unknown, but it is often quoted in discussions of Hebbian learning in neuroscience. See J. L. McClelland, "How Far Can You Go with Hebbian Learning, and When Does It Lead you Astray?" available at www.psych.stanford.edu/~jlm/papers/McClellandIPHowFar.pdf.

50   **this capacity of our brains to impose order and meaning:** Anticipation can affect perception. There has been much research by Nancy Kanwisher and her team at MIT to show how, by directing our attention, we can alter what we perceive of our environment. "We are not passive recipients but active participants in our own process of perception." N. Kanwisher and P. Downing, 1998, "Separating the Wheat from the Chaff," *Science* 282:57–58.

55   **mouths that do not speak:** Psalms 135:16–17 (New American Standard Bible).

58–59   **"We now know that with proper stimulation and an enriched environment":** M. Diamond, from a lecture to the American Society on Aging, 2001, quoted in D. Amen, 2005, *Making a Good Brain Great* (New York: Harmony Books), 113.

61   **our brains switch on and create something new:** Constantine Mangina and Evgeni Sokolov have distinguished two kinds of intelligence in terms of the potential to acquire knowledge. The first, *crystallized intelligence,* is fact-based intelligence (academic learning) and is the intelligence mostly focused on by traditional education. The second one, *fluid intelligence,* operates under novel situations and is responsible for the acquisition of new information (organic learning). They claim that fluid intelligence reaches its peak at around twenty-five years of age and gradually declines thereafter if left on its own (but see below). They defined "optimally high" physiological activation in the brain during which fluid intelligence occurs (i.e., the learning switch is turned on). C. A. Mangina and E. N. Sokolov, 2006, "Neuronal Plasticity in Memory and Learning Difficulties: Theoretical Position and Selective Review," *International Journal of Psychophysiology* 60:203–214.

Michael Merzenich has identified the role of a subcortical structure in the brain called the basal nucleus. During infant development, it is very active, but its level of activity tends to go down in later years. When it is reactivated in later life, adults become better learners. In other words, the ability for organic learning is not lost, just dormant. M. P. Kilgard and M. M. Merzenich, 1998, "Cortical Map Reorganization Enabled by Nucleus Basalis Activity," *Science* 279(5357):1714–1718.

A new study from the University of Michigan appears to show that fluid intelligence is *not* innate. The kind of mental ability that allows us to solve new problems without having any relevant experience is a skill that can be trained. S. M. Jaeggi, M. Buschkuehl, J. Jonides, and W. J. Perrig, 2008, "Improving Fluid Intelligence with Training on Working Memory," *Proceedings of the National Academy of Sciences* 105(19):6829–6833. See also N. Balakar, 2008, "Memory Training Shown to Turn Up Brainpower," *New York Times* April 29.

70   **an inevitable offshoot of civilization's demands on us:** S. Freud, *Civilization and Its Discontents* (New York: W. W. Norton).

71   **how we handle stress in our lives can either empower us or tranquilize us:** A. Patmore, 2006, *The Truth About Stress* (London: Atlantic Books).

72   **" 'flow'—that wonderful state":** R. Gross, "Your Learning and Your Brain," available at http://adulted.about.com/od/learningstyles/a/brain_2.htm.

74   **Roger Bannister, the man who, in 1954, broke the four-minute mile, was surrounded by scientists "proving" the human body was not capable of breaking the four-minute mile:** Bannister himself discusses this and believes that the notion of the impossibility of a four-minute mile may have been a myth created by sportswriters and not the view of contemporary experts. R. Bannister, 2004, *The Four-Minute Mile*, rev. ed. (Guildford, CT: Lyons Press)

76   **"the finest work of literature in all the annals of science . . .":** P. B. Medawar, quoted in J. T. Bonner's editorial introduction to the Canto edition of D. Thompson, 1961, *On Growth and Form* (Cambridge: Cambridge University Press), xv.

THREE. SUBTLETY—EXPERIENCE THE POWER OF GENTLENESS

83   **we begin to notice finer differences:** Jay McLelland, of Stanford University, used a computer to exaggerate the phonetic distinctions between "l" and "r" that normally confuse Japanese speakers.

McLelland enabled the Japanese adults to perceive the differences between the two sounds more easily. They thus learned to be able to recognize and reproduce the sounds. B. D. McCandliss, J. A. Fiez, A. Protopapas, M. Conway, and J. L. McClelland, 2002, "Success and Failure in Teaching the [r]-[l] Contrast to Japanese Adults: Predictions of a Hebbian Model of Plasticity and Stabilization in Spoken Language Perception," *Cognitive, Affective and Behavioral Neuroscience* 2:89–108.

84   **A scientist and rehabilitation physician by the name of Paul Bach-y-Rita:** See N. Doidge, 2007, *The Brain That Changes Itself: Stories of Personal Triumph from the Frontiers of Brain Science* (New York: Viking Penguin), 19–20. Bach-y-Rita extended his exploration to substituting tactile stimulation for other sensory modalities, most notably and extraordinarily with vision, realizing that "we see with the brain and not the eyes." P. Bach-y-Rita, M. E. Tyler, and K. A. Kaczmarek, 2003, "Seeing with the Brain," *International Journal of Human-Computer Interaction* 15(2):285–295; P. Bach-y-Rita, J. G. Webster, W. J. Tompkins, and T. Crab, 1987, "Sensory Substitution for Space Gloves and Space Robots," Space Telerobotics Workshop, Jet Propulsion Laboratory, Pasadena, Calif., January 20–22, 51–57.

96   **Ernst Heinrich Weber showed:** Weber's finding, known as the Weber-Fechner law, is mainly founded on experiments in which people were given two nearly identical stimuli (for example, two similar weights) and tested whether they could notice a difference between them. It was found that the smallest noticeable difference was roughly proportional to the intensity of the stimulus. For example, if a person could consistently feel that a 110-gram weight was heavier than a 100-gram weight, he could also feel that 1,100 grams was more than 1,000 grams.

More recently, it has become evident that the Weber-Fechner principle applies mainly to higher intensities of sight, hearing, and touch and only poorly to most other types of sensory experience. However, the Weber-Fechner principle is still a good one to remember because it emphasizes that the greater the intensity of the background sensory stimulus, the harder it is to perceive a change. See www.neuro.uu.se/fysiologi/gu/nbb/lectures/WebFech.html and A. C. Guyton, 1981, *Textbook of Medical Physiology* (Philadelphia: Saunders).

104   **the story of Juan Fangio:** The story of the crash and Fangio's subsequent realization is to be found in D. Kim Rossmo, 2006,

"Criminal Investigative Failures," *FBI—Law Enforcement Bulletin* 75(9):1–10.

Four. Variation—Enjoy Abundant Possibilities

108 A group of brain researchers asked if physical activity alone: J. E. Black, K. R. Isaacs, B. J. Anderson, A. A. Alcantara, and W. T. Greenough, 1990, "Learning Causes Synaptogenesis, Whereas Motor Activity Causes Angiogenesis, in Cerebellar Cortex of Adult Rats," *Proceedings of the National Academy of Sciences* 87:5568–5572.

111 "motor skill is not a movement formula": N. A. Bernstein, 1996, "On Exercise and Motor Skill," in *On Dexterity and Its Development,* translated by M. L. Latash, ed. M. L. Latash and M. T. Tuvey (Mahwah, NJ: Lawrence Erlbaum), 181.

111 In an article titled "The Plastic Human Brain Cortex": A. Pascual-Leone, A. Amedi, F. Fregni, and L. B. Merabet, 2005, "The Plastic Human Brain Cortex," *Annual Reviews of Neuroscience* 28:380.

112 "We are just beginning to realize that the adult brain is more dynamic than static": M. M. Mezernich, J. H. Kaas, J. T. Wall, R. J. Nelson, M. Sur, and D. Felleman, 1983, "Topographic Reorganization of Somatosensory Cortical Areas 3B and 1 in Adult Monkeys Following Restricted Deafferentation," *Neuroscience* 8:33–55.

120 "By our errors we see deeper into life." From the novel *The Story of an African Farm,* published in 1883 by the South African novelist, pacifist, and social critic Olive Emilie Albertino Schreiner under her pseudonym Ralph Iron.

120 the sensory receptors—the nerve cells through which we experience all sensations—"react strongly while change is taking place": A. C. Guyton, 1981, *Textbook of Medical Physiology* (Philadelphia: Saunders).

120 the often-told story of Friedrich Kekulé: Kekulé himself recounted the anecdote in a speech to the German Chemical Society in 1890, some twenty-five years after publishing his theory. See A. J. Rocke, 1985, "Hypothesis and Experiment in the Early Development of Kekulé's Benzene Theory," *Annals of Science* 42:4, 355–381.

124 To get rid of the pain: See chapter 1.

130 William Westney, a concert pianist and award-winning educator: See W. Westney, 2006, *The Perfect Wrong Note: Learning to Trust Your Musical Self* (Pompton Plains, NJ: Amadeus Press), 156.

131   "To fall into a habit is to begin to cease to be": M. de Unamuno, 2007, *Del Sentimiento Trágico de la Vida (The Tragic Sense of Life)* (Milano, Italy: Dodo Press), chap. 9.

Five. Slow—Luxuriate in the Richness of Feeling

136   **Scientific research shows that we can either react automatically with a shorter reaction time of 0.25 seconds or less, or act consciously with a delayed reaction time of 0.5 seconds or more:** In a series of extraordinary and elegant experiments, Benjamin Libet has shown that electrical activity in the brain, called "the readiness potential," precedes our awareness of a consciously willed action by about 0.5 seconds—that is, the brain starts an action half a second *before* we *decide* to act! If this action is in response to a stimulus, the awareness occurs half a second after the stimulus, but the subjective conscious experience is projected back in time closer to the moment of the stimulus (0.02 seconds after, in fact).

So it takes a little time for us to perceive the outside world, but we relocate the experience back in time so that we experience the world at the right moment.

Arthur Jensen carried out a series of reaction-time experiments in the 1960s in which subjects demonstrated reaction times of about 0.25 seconds. He wondered if some of the subjects were cheating by deliberately being too slow, so he asked them to gradually increase their reaction time, but none of them could. As soon as they tried to increase their reaction time to more than a quarter of a second, it leaped to at least half a second—a result that was explained by Libet's findings.

So, things that need to happen quickly happen automatically. For us to have a conscious say in our actions, we need to act a lot more slowly. Libet's findings are discussed extensively in T. Norretranders, 1998, *The User Illusion: Cutting Consciousness Down to Size* (New York: Viking Penguin), chaps. 9, 10, and 11. His writings are based on an interview with Libet on March 26 and 27, 1991, in San Francisco. See also B. Libet et al., 1983, "Time of Conscious Intention to Act in Relation to Onset of Cerebral Activity (Readiness Potential): The Unconscious Intention of a Freely Voluntary Act," *Brain* 106:623–642.

137   **Slow gets the brain's attention, increasing its activity and forming new patterns:** Jeffrey Schwartz is a psychologist who specializes in treating the debilitating condition of obsessive-compulsive disorder

(OCD). He describes an OCD "circuit" in the brain that becomes chronically and inappropriately activated and has developed a four-step treatment regime that is informed by his practices in Buddhist meditation. Slowing down and paying attention provide a "way in" to disturb these harmful patterns and enable the formation of newer healthier ones. He says, "Directed mental focusing of attention becomes the mind's key action during treatment." J. M. Schwartz and S. Begley, 2003, *The Mind and the Brain: Neuroplasticity and the Power of Mental Force* (New York: ReganBooks), 55–95, 338–340.

138   **In her book *You Are Not the Target*, . . . Laura Archera Huxley:** L. Archera Huxley, 1995. (Portland, OR: Metamorphons Press).

139–140   **"Having someone wonder where you are when you don't come home at night is a very old human need":** Margaret Mead, from a speech published in M. Brown and A. O'Connor, 1985, *Woman Talk* (London: Futura Publications).

140   **In his book *Flow*:** M. Csikszentmihalyi, 1990, *Flow: The Psychology of Optimal Experience* (New York: Harper Perennial).

140   **"freed from normal restrictions, and are opened to a wider world":** Madeleine L'Engle, 1980, *Walking on Water: Reflections on Faith and Art.*

141   **Intentionally slowing down can help us perceive differences:** Paula Tallal and Michael Merzenich developed a program for children with language learning impairment called Fast ForWord, which slows down the sounds that children hear, allowing them to begin to distinguish between the sounds and overcome their limitations. P. Tallal, 1998, "Language Learning Impairment: Integrating Research and Remediation," *New Horizons for Learning.* http://www.newhorizons.org/neuro/tallal/htm.

151   **Slow is for creation and learning:** To master anything we do, we need initially to slow way down, and then we can speed up successfully and even develop strong intuition in that area. D. Kahnman, 2003, "A Perspective on Judgement and Choice: Mapping Bounded Rationality," *American Psychologist* 58:697–720.

Six. Enthusiasm—Turn the Small into the Great

157   **Enthusiasm can have a powerful impact on our moods, our behavior, and our physical performance:** Enthusiasm amplifies our experience, and amplification is a characteristic of many biological systems for example, our senses of taste and smell. Taste and

(even more especially) smell are characterized by a very low sensory threshold. One of the principle characteristics of smell is the minute quantity of the stimulating agent in the air often required to effect a smell sensation. For instance, the substance methyl mercaptan can be smelled when only 1/25,000,000,000 milligram is present in each milliliter of air. Because of this low threshold, this substance is mixed with natural gas to give it an odor that can be detected when it leaks from a gas pipe. A. C. Guyton, 1981, *Textbook of Medical Physiology* (Saunders).

Through this process of amplification, one molecule of a fragrant flower can lead us to remember an old friend and travel across the world to visit her.

157 **"we can think of emotions, moods and states such as compassion as trainable mental skills":** A. Lutz, L. L. Greischar, N. B. Rawlings, and R. Davidson, 2004, "Long-Term Meditators Self-Induce High-Amplitude Gamma Synchrony During Mental Practice," *Proceedings of the National Academy of Sciences* 101(46):16369–16373.

160 **every time he noted a change he liked and amplified it internally:** In his book *Looking for Spinoza: Joy, Sorrow and the Feeling Brain,* 2003, internationally renowned neuroscientist Antonio Damasio argued that the mind and body are unified. He anticipated one of brain science's most important recent discoveries: the critical role of the emotions in ensuring our survival and allowing us to think. See E. Eakin, 2003, "I Feel Therefore I Am," *New York Times,* April 19.

Current research and theory point ever more clearly to the link between our emotions and our brain's ability and tendency to learn, remember, and create new patterns and possibilities for us. Positive anticipation is shown to play an important role in these domains. S. Ikemoto and J. Panksepp, 1999, "The Role of Nucleus Accumbens Dopamine in Motivated Behavior: A Unifying Interpretation with Special Reference to Reward-Seeking," *Brain Research Reviews* 31(1):6–41.

167 **This spontaneous excitement essentially gets her brain to pay attention and select the relevant connections that are being formed and to make sure to strengthen those connections:** An emotionally arousing stimulus places the brain in a "motive state," coordinating information processing across the brain and leading to invigoration. Animals become active or invigorated when dopamine is injected into a particular area in the forebrain called

the nucleus accumbens. Dopamine facilitates synaptic transmission, leading to amplification in circuits that lead to activation of movement-control regions. Novel stimuli and incentives are prime examples of invigorating stimuli. J. LeDoux, 2002, *Synaptic Self: How Our Brains Become Who We Are* (New York: Viking Penguin), 243–259.

172   **When we are without enthusiasm, we miss out on a powerful tool:** One of the periods of greatest enthusiasm and change in adult life is when we fall in love. Oxytocin is a neuromodulator (a chemical that enhances or diminishes the overall effectiveness of nerve transmission at synapses) that is released when lovers commit. One of its roles seems to be the "wiping out" of neural patterns, making it possible for the couple to learn new ones. The work of Walter Freeman, a professor of neuroscience at the University of California, Berkeley, in this area is discussed in N. Doidge, 2007, *The Brain That Changes Itself* (New York: Viking Penguin), 118–121.

172   **When Winnie-the-Pooh found Eeyore's lost tail:** A. A. Milne, 1926, *Winnie-the-Pooh* (London: Methuen), chap. 4, "When Eeyore Lost a Tail, and Pooh Found One."

173   **"offered strong evidence that willful, mindful effort can alter brain function":** J. M. Schwartz, P. W. Stoessel, L. R. Baxter Jr., K. M. Martin, and M. E. Phelps, 1996, "Systematic Changes in Cerebral Glucose Metabolic Rate After Successful Behavior Modification Treatment of Obsessive-Compulsive Disorder," *Archives of General Psychiatry* 53:109–113.

176   **"Moment by moment we choose and sculpt how our ever changing minds will work":** M. M. Merzenich and R. C. Decharms, 1996, "Neural Representations, Experience and Change," in *The Mind-Brain Continuum*, ed. R. Llinàs and P. S. Churchland (Cambridge, MA: MIT Press), 61–81.

177   **All things in the universe move toward states of greater *entropy*:** The concept of entropy in physics is a measure of the degree of order of a particular system. It is a quantity that, in principle, can be calculated. Increased entropy means loss of order. The entropy of an *isolated* system always increases; for example, leave your backyard furniture outdoors for the duration of a New England winter and see what happens to the shape and color of the cushions. Or leave your brain unattended for a couple of decades and experience increased entropy in your mind and body firsthand! However, the trend in any particular system can be reversed and

moved toward greater order, popularly known as *negative* entropy. For example, order can be increased by cooling a liquid to make it solidify, or, more spectacularly, by humans building high-rise office blocks out of sand and cement or violins out of chunks of wood. It is important to note, however, that order is not the same as complexity, and it is in the realm of complexity that we talk about order in the brain. "Complexity covers a vast territory that lies between order and chaos." H. Pagels, 1989, *The Dreams of Reason: The Computer and the Rise of the Sciences of Complexity* (New York: Bantam), 66.

We will return to complexity in chapter 11.

Order and information are also linked, although, once again, they are not the same. For example, a crystal contains much order but little information, whereas a gas lacks order but its particles represent a lot of information as noise. What is important is the value, or meaning, that it is possible to extract from that information.

It is easy to appreciate how misconceptions have arisen in this complex and challenging field when the father of information theory himself is quoted as saying the following regarding the concept of entropy:

> My greatest concern was what to call it. I thought of calling it "information," but the word was overly used, so I decided to call it "uncertainty." When I discussed it with John von Neumann, he had a better idea. Von Neumann told me, "You should call it entropy, for two reasons. In the first place your uncertainty function has been used in statistical mechanics under that name, so it already has a name. In the second place, and more important, nobody knows what entropy really is, so in a debate you will always have the advantage."

From a conversation between Claude Shannon and John von Neumann regarding what name to give to the "measure of uncertainty" or attenuation in phone-line signals (1949). Quoted in M. Tribus and E. C. McIrvine, 1971. "Energy and Information." *Scientific American* 224(3):179–188.

For an in-depth discussion of information, meaning, depth, and entropy, see T. Norretranders, 1998, *The User Illusion: Cutting Consciousness Down to Size* (New York: Viking Penguin).

177 Another example is the way a flower dies and soon disintegrates: Noted American biochemist Albert Lehninger has argued that the order produced within cells as they grow and divide is more than compensated for by the disorder they create in their surroundings in the course of growth and division: ". . . living organisms preserve their internal order . . . returning to their surroundings an equal amount of energy as heat and entropy." A. Lehringer, 1993, *Principles of Biochemistry, 2nd ed.* (New York: Worth).

SEVEN. FLEXIBLE GOALS—MAKE THE IMPOSSIBLE POSSIBLE

183 by holding our goals loosely: Goal-setting theory has been popular in organizational psychology. Edwin A. Locke began to examine this subject in the mid-1960s and derived the concept for goal setting from the work of the Greek philosopher Aristotle. According to Aristotle, action is caused by a purpose. There are limitations to goal-setting theory, and for complex tasks, an individual may become preoccupied with meeting the goals, rather than performing the task, thereby impairing performance. G. Latham, E. Locke, 2002, "Building a Practically Useful Theory of Goal Setting and Task Motivation: A 35-Year Odyssey," *American Psychologist* 57(9):705–717.

183 In the documentary film *Animals Are Beautiful People:* Written, produced, and directed by J. Uys, distributed by Warner Bros., 1975.

185 the Chicago Columbus Day marathon: A. Wang, 2007, "One Dead in Heat-Shortened Marathon," *Chicago Tribune*, October 7.

186 We even carry our rigid approach to goal setting into raising our children: Students do better when they focus on becoming proficient rather than on achieving grades. They engage with the task more deeply and persevere in the face of setbacks.

If their focus is on good grades as a mark of success, these become the indicators of self-worth, and this goal-orientated approach is associated with higher anxiety and an increased tendency to cheat or learn by rote, rather than striving for a deeper understanding. C. Ames, 1992, "Achievement Goals, Motivational Climate and Motivational Processes," in *Motivation in Sport and Exercise,* ed. G. C. Roberts (Human Kinetics: Champaign, IL.) 161–176.

188   In his award-winning book *Ever Since Darwin:* S. J. Gould, 2007, *Ever Since Darwin* (New York: W. W. Norton), 68.

189   **At birth, our brains are roughly a quarter of their adult size:** "At birth, the brain of a rhesus monkey is 65 percent of its final size, a chimpanzee's is 40.5 percent, but we attain only 23 percent. Chimps and gorillas reach 70 percent of final brain size early in their first year; we do not achieve this value until early in our third year. W. M. Krogman, our leading expert in child growth, has written: 'Man has absolutely the most protracted period of infancy, childhood and juvenility of all forms of life . . . Nearly 30 percent of his life is devoted to growing.' " Ibid.

189   **"Play is the best way to reach certain goals":** Bateson is quoted in R. Marantz Henig, 2008, "Why Do We Play?" *New York Times Magazine*, February 17.

189   **Instead, we are able to respond to the present, where our brains best perform their creative magic:** Inflexibility of approach is seen at its extreme in patients with obsessive-compulsive disorder (OCD). Current research shows that people suffering from obsessive-compulsive disorder have certain circuits in their brains that keep getting activated, usually by a fear or an anxiety that is created within their brain with no direct correlation to events in the world outside their brain. J. M. Schwartz and S. Begley, 2003, *The Mind and the Brain: Neuroplasticity and the Power of Mental Force* (New York: ReganBooks), 61–65.

Psychologist Jeffrey Schwartz has developed mindfulness techniques to help people overcome these limiting patterns of thought. Release from these obsessive thought patterns "also results in an extremely rewarding sense of true self-esteem—that empowering inner awareness that the utilization of knowledge has enhanced one's capacity for self-control." J. M. Schwartz, 1999, "A Role for Volition and Attention in the Generation of New Brain Circuitry—Toward a Neurobiology of Mental Force." *Journal of Consciousness Studies* 6(8–9):115–142.

190   **Some of the most creative musicians, artists, and scientists have experienced the benefits:** Stuart Brown, president of the National Institute for Play, is quoted as saying: "If you look at what produces learning and memory and well-being, play is as fundamental as any other aspect of life, including sleep and dreams." Henig, "Why Do We Play?"

190   **Wolfgang Amadeus Mozart once reflected:** This quotation is from a letter published by Friedrich Rochlitz in the *Allgemeine*

Musikalische Zeitung in 1815 (17:561–566) and purported to be by Mozart. A surviving letter of Mozart's to his father, Leopold, (July 31, 1778) indicates that he considered composition to be an active rather than a passive process: "You know that I immerse myself in music, so to speak—that I think about it all day long—that I like experimenting—studying—reflecting." U. Konrad, 2005, "Compositional Method," in *The Cambridge Mozart Encyclopedia,* ed. C. Eisen and S. P. Keefe (Cambridge, U.K.: Cambridge University Press), 101.

195   In his book *The Farther Reaches of Human Nature,* Maslow said: A. Maslow, 1971, *The Farther Reaches of Human Nature* (New York: Viking).

196   "The test of a first-rate intelligence": F. Scott Fitzgerald, 1936, *The Crack-Up.* (New York: New Directions Publishing Corp.).

203   In a recent *New York Times* article, author Gary Rivlin profiled Max Levchin: G. Rivlin, 2007, "Age of Riches: After Succeeding, Young Tycoons Try, Try Again," *New York Times,* October 28.

204   As Stephen Jay Gould claims: Gould, *Ever Since Darwin,* 73.

204   Recently, Nobel Prize winner Oliver Smithies, a geneticist, was interviewed: C. Lee, 2007, "From Child on Street to Nobel Laureate," *Washington Post,* October 9, A01.

EIGHT. IMAGINATION AND DREAMS—CREATE YOUR LIFE

208   In a study of how our brains operate during normal day-to-day activities: M. F. Mason, M. I. Norton, J. D. Van Horn, D. M. Wegner, S. T. Grafton, and C. N. Macrae, 2007, "Wandering Minds: The Default Network and Stimulus-Independent Thought," *Science* 315 (5810):393–395. Reported in H. Jones, 2007, "Daydreaming Improves Thinking," *Cosmos Online,* January 19. http://www.cosmosmagazine.com/node/980.

208   In another study of six thousand men and women: S. J. Lynn and J. W. Rhue, 1988, "Fantasy Proneness: Hypnosis, Developmental Antecedents, and Psychopathology," *American Psychologist* 43(1):35–44.

209   during sleep, different areas of our brains talk to each other: D. Y. Ji and M. A. Wilson, 2007, "Coordinated Memory Replay in the Visual Cortex and Hippocampus During Sleep," *Nature Neuroscience* 10:100–107, reported in B. Carey, 2007, "An Active, Purposeful Machine That Comes Out at Night to Play: Some Neuroscientists Say That at Least One Vital Function of Sleep Is

Tied to Learning and Memory, and New Findings Suggest That Sleep Plays a Crucial Role in Flagging and Storing Important Memories," *New York Times,* October 23.

211 **In research conducted by Alvaro Pascual-Leone:** Pascual-Leone and his colleagues say that

> mental practice alone led to the same plastic changes in the motor system as those occurring with the acquisition of the skill by repeated physical practice. . . . Mental practice alone seems to be sufficient to promote the modulation of neural circuits involved in the early stages of motor skill learning. This modulation not only results in marked performance improvement, but also seems to place the subjects at an advantage for further skill learning with minimal physical practice.

They were literally thinking themselves into a new brain. A. Pascual-Leone, D. Nguyet, L. G. Cohen, J. P. Brasil-Neto, A. Cammarota, and M. Hallett, 1995, "Modulation of Muscle Responses Evoked by Transcranial Magnetic Stimulation During the Acquisition of New Fine Motor Skills," *Journal of Neurophysiology* 74:1037–1045. For a review of his research with functional MRI imaging from the study, see also A. Pascual-Leone, A. Amedi, F. Fregni, and L. B. Merabet, 2005, "The Plastic Human Brain Cortex," *Annual Revue of Neuroscience* 28:377–401.

217 **In an interesting study published in *Psychological Science*:** A. J. Crum and E. J. Langer, 2007, "Mind-Set Matters: Exercise and the Placebo Effect," *Psychological Science* 18(2):165–171.

220 **In Marty Klein's book *Beyond Orgasm*:** M. Klein, 2002, *Beyond Orgasm* (San Francisco, CA: Celestial Arts).

222 **Most of us have heard the famous speech of Martin Luther King Jr.:** Delivered on August 28, 1963, at the Lincoln Memorial in Washington, D.C., as part of the March on Washington for Jobs and Freedom. The speech marked a pivotal point in the American civil rights movement.

224 **"Your health is bound to be affected if, day after day, you say the opposite of what you feel":** B. Pasternak, 1958, *Dr. Zhivago.* (New York: Pantheon Books).

224 **Joseph Campbell, who coined the phrase "follow your bliss":** See J. Campbell with B. Moyers and B. S. Flowers, ed., 1988, *The Power of Myth* (New York: Doubleday), 117.

224   "People who follow a dream or have a deep sense of purpose":
       D. Jaffe and C. Scott, 1988, *Take This Job and Love It* (New
       York: Fireside).

225   Bestselling author Gary Zukav calls it our "authentic power":
       G. Zukav, 1997, *Authentic Power: Aligning Personality with Soul*
       (Carlsbad, CA: Hay House Audio Books).

225   And it is what Henry David Thoreau was reflecting on: H. D.
       Thoreau, 1989, *Walden; or, Life in the Woods* (Princeton, N.J.:
       Princeton University Press).

225   Abraham Maslow saw these visions and dreams in a similar
       light: A. Maslow, 1998, *Toward a Psychology of Being*, 3rd ed.
       (New York: Wiley).

225   "You gotta have a dream": Lyrics from the song "Happy Talk,"
       from *South Pacific*, 1949, music by Richard Rodgers and lyrics by
       Oscar Hammerstein II.

231   skeptics flourish, ready to proclaim the impossibility of whatever
       new ideas are being put forth: The great contemporary neurosci-
       entist V. S. Ramachandran is passionate about how important it is
       for science to embrace and investigate phenomena that are too fre-
       quently dismissed because, for example, there is not enough statis-
       tical evidence. V. S. Ramachandran, 2006, "Creativity Versus
       Skepticism Within Science: More Harm Has Been Done in Science
       by Those Who Make a Fetish out of Skepticism, Aborting Ideas
       Before They Are Born, Than by Those Who Gullibly Accept
       Untested Theories," *Skeptical Inquirer* 30(6):48–51.

232   On October 9, 1903, for example, the *New York Times:* From
       J. Carreau, 2007, "The Invincible Man—Aubrey de Grey,
       44 Going on 1,000, Wants Out of Old Age," *Washington Post*,
       October 31, C01.

NINE. AWARENESS—THRIVE WITH TRUE KNOWLEDGE

235   Awareness is different from attention: On a neurological level,
       attention can be seen as a combination of sensory processing
       and working memory. It is a selection process whereby some
       stimuli are processed more efficiently than others; for example, a
       moving stimulus is perceived more readily than a stationary one.
       The complexity of the connections between nerve cells is so
       great that even the fundamental properties that explain the rela-
       tionship between perception and action still evade us; however,
       enough is known for us to imagine, in principle, how this might

occur. In addition, memory can be understood in basic terms of the plasticity of the connections between nerve cells in response to experience.

Awareness, on the other hand, relates to the highest levels of consciousness, for which there are as yet no clear known neural correlates. Part of what needs to be explained is how different aspects of perceived stimuli become "bound" together, and then how we become aware of them when they do. Victor Lamme suggests that the binding results from interactions of groups of neurons, which may grow more widespread and come to include higher centers of the brain involved in so-called executive functions. They are put into the context of the system's current needs, goals, and full history. They may thereby reach awareness. V. A. Lamme, 2003, "Why Visual Attention and Awareness Are Different," *Trends in Cognitive Neurosciences* 7(1):12–18; V. A. Lamme, 2004, "Separate Neural Definitions of Visual Consciousness and Visual Attention: A Case for Phenomenal Awareness," *Neural Networks* 17(5–6):861–72. Department of Psychology, University of Amsterdam.

235   **Awareness, as I use the term here, means knowing that you know:** There is a good reason for defining the term so specifically. Until very recently, consciousness and awareness were the domain of philosophers. With the explosion of knowledge from brain research in the past two decades, it has become a legitimate area for exploration by neuroscientists; but such exploration is still in its infancy, and definitions remain vague. Christof Koch, one of the world's leading cognitive neuroscientists, writes in his recent book, *The Quest for Consciousness,* "Throughout the book, I use *awareness* and *consciousness* as synonyms." C. Koch, 2004, *The Quest for Consciousness: A Neurobiological Approach* (Englewood, Colo.: Roberts), 12 n19.

Eleanor Rosch, a professor in the Department of Psychology at the University of California at Berkeley, acknowledged the difficulties the concept of awareness presents to science in a conversation with the Dalai Lama.

Dalai Lama: "Now, from the point of view of a Western psychologist, how would you prove the presence of something called awareness, the instrument of knowledge?" Rosch: "Well, you see, that is exactly what Western psychologists do not know how to demonstrate."

J. W. Hayward and F. J. Varela, eds., 2001, *Gentle Bridges: Conversations with the Dalai Lama on the Sciences of Mind* (Boston: Shambhala), 116.

I chose to use the word *awareness* exclusively because I distinguish it from *consciousness*, which is a state during which one could, for example, walk through a door without his body hitting the door frame but not necessarily be aware of it.

235 **Other animals have some rudimentary consciousness:** The high level of awareness whereby we have an internal observer of ourselves and those around us that knows what it knows seems to be a capacity of the human mind alone, although there is much evidence that limited consciousness exists in many animal species and that "some monkeys even know what they know." D. R. Griffin and G. B. Speck, 2004, "New Evidence of Animal Consciousness," *Journal of Animal Cognition* 7(1):5–18.

237 **Perceiving a stimulus and even reacting to it does not mean that we are aware of it at all:** Although there has been much debate over the phenomenon of subliminal perception, "there is considerable evidence for perception without awareness. In fact it is relatively easy to demonstrate that perception occurs when subjects do not believe they have either seen or heard an adequate stimulus." P. M. Meirikle, 1992, "Perception Without Awareness. Critical Issues," *American Psychologist* 47(6):792–795.

One striking example of perception without awareness is known as *blindsight*. Some brain-damaged patients claim to be blind yet perform tasks that seem impossible unless they can see. "In a sense we all suffer from blindsight," says V. S. Ramachandran, who uses the example given in this text of driving while deeply engaged in conversation. V. S. Ramachandran, 2003, *The Emerging Mind: The Reith Lectures, 2003* (London: Profile Books), 182. See also F. C. Kolb and J. Braun, 1995, "Blindsight in Normal Observers," *Nature* 377:336–338.

237 **Without awareness, we could move our shoulder or arm thousands of times:** Dick Passingham and his colleagues compared new learning and subsequent automatic performance in normal volunteers using PET scans. The scans showed particular metabolic activity during new learning but not during automatic performance. When asked to become aware of the now-automatic task, the silent brain became metabolically active once more. M. Jueptner, K. M. Stephan, C. D. Frith, D. J. Brooks, R. S. J. Frackowiak, and R. E. Passingham, 1997, "Anatomy of Motor Learning: I. Frontal

Cortex and Attention to Action," *Journal of Neurophysiology* 77(3):1313–1324.

237–238 **Whether those automatic behaviors serve us well or not:** Habits are undoubtedly important. Cristof Koch talks about our having a number of stereotyped behaviors, or *zombie agents,* that bypass consciousness. Initial acquisition of these *zombie agents* requires awareness, and then we operate by a combination of these learned automatic responses and a slower but more-flexible conscious response to a situation. Koch, *Quest for Consciousness,* 231–247.

The important thing is to be able to learn something new. "Brain researchers have discovered that when we consciously develop new habits, we create parallel synaptic paths, and even entirely new brain cells, that can jump our trains of thought onto new innovative tracks." J. Rae-Dupree, 2008, "Can You Become a Creature of New Habits?" *New York Times,* May 4.

238 **once we become aware of it, knowledge rushes in:** Jueptner, et al. "Anatomy of Motor Learning," 1313–1324.

238 **awareness in one person can bring about a shift in another:** In the social sciences, the term *Hawthorne effect* refers to how people change their behavior when aware of being watched. The Hawthorne effect gets its name from the Hawthorne Works factory in Chicago, where a series of experiments on factory workers were carried out between 1924 and 1932. Although the results are now questionable, the term has come to be used to describe the phenomenon in which being observed by another can and often will shift our behavior. S. R. G. Jones, 1992, "Was There a Hawthorne Effect?" *American Journal of Sociology* 98(3):451–468.

In science, the term *observer effect* refers to the effect that the act of observation will have on the phenomenon being observed. Jeffrey Schwartz writes, "Quantum physics makes the seemingly preposterous claim (. . . upheld in countless experiments) that there is no 'is' until an observer makes an observation." Until something is observed, it is a "quantum smear" of potential for the occurrence of various possible observed feedbacks. Schwartz has collaborated with Henry Stapp, a physicist at Lawrence Berkeley National Laboratory at University of California at Berkeley. Stapp sees no justification for those quantum physicists who base neuroscience on classical physics by suggesting that once brain activity reaches the level of, say, the firing of a neuron, this quantum jump from possible to actual has occurred. He argues first for quantum principles of uncertainty at synapses and then extends this to the behavior of the whole brain. In this context, the observer and the observed are each "a smeared out continuum of classically conceivable possibilities," with the observed being partitioned into a set of discrete components by an agent who is himself a continuous smear of possibilities! Stapp's controversial ideas are discussed in chapters 8 through 10 of J. M. Schwartz and S. Begley, 2002, *The Mind and the Brain: Neuroplasticity and the Power of Mental Force* (New York: ReganBooks). See also H. P. Stapp, 2007, *Mindful Universe: Quantum Mechanics and the Participating Observer* (Berlin: Springer-Verlag).

241 **Awareness requires the capacity for the observation of self and others:** The human brain has an observational capacity *built in.* In the 1980s, Giacomo Rizzolatti and his colleagues identified a type of brain cell he termed a *mirror neuron.* Present in humans and some other primates, they fire when observing the actions of another. Mirror neurons in themselves, of course, do not explain the highly complex processes behind awareness. Giacomo Rizzolatti et al., 1996, "Premotor Cortex and the Recognition of Motor Actions," *Cognitive Brain Research* 3:131–141.

242 **she becomes aware of herself in a new way:** Other research extends this mirror system (see note above) beyond merely seeing an action; that is, they are responsible for more than just *monkey see, monkey do.* "Any sensorial cue that can evoke the 'idea' of a meaningful action activates the vocabulary of motor representations." Moreover, they are thought to be key in the learning of language, empathy, and emotions. L. Craighero, G. Metta, G. Sandini, and L. Fadiga, 2007, "The Mirror-Neurons System: Data and Models," in *From Action to Cognition,* ed. Claes Von Hofsten and Kerstin Rosander, vol. 164 of Progress in Brain Research (St. Louis, MO: Elsevier), 39–59.

243 **Awareness, like movement, is something that we do—or not:** Awareness as an action has been practiced and developed for centuries in the Buddhist tradition and is now the subject of intense scientific scrutiny. Researchers are studying the impact of meditation practices, which involve intense self-observation, on brain plasticity and performance. M. Barinaga, 2003, "Buddhism and Neuroscience: Studying the Well-Trained Mind," *Science* 302(5642):44–46.

MOVE INTO LIFE

254   **a process called *differentiation*:** K. N. Prasad, 1980, *Regulation of Differentiation in Mammalian Nerve Cells.* (New York: Plenum) 2–3.

254   **Scientists are able to measure and track the process of differentiation as it is taking place in the brain:** Dr. Adi Mizrahi, of the Department of Neurobiology at the Alexander Silberman Institute of Life Sciences at the Hebrew University, used time-lapse photography to study how mouse nerve cells develop from an undifferentiated cellular sphere into a rich and complex cell. "The structural and functional complexity of nerve cells remains one of the biggest mysteries of neuroscience, and we now have a model to study this complexity directly," he said. "Scientist Observes Brain Cell Development in 'Real Time.'" *ScienceDaily,* May 29, 2007; A. Mizrahi, 2007, "Dendritic Development and Plasticity of Adult-Born Neurons in the Mouse Olfactory Bulb," *Nature Neuroscience* 10(4):444–452.

254   **as we gain a new skill, or improve on an existing one, more brain cells get involved:** When we begin to learn a new skill, such as riding a bike, our initial clumsy efforts result from the use of too much unrefined muscular effort. We are unable to make subtle adjustments in response to the movement of the bike and the pull of the gravitational force, so we fall. As we gain experience, we gain control through using our muscles in a more refined and precise way. This process has been demonstrated in the brain. William Jenkins and Michael Merzenich trained monkeys to touch a spinning disk with one of their fingertips and then mapped their sensory cortex. The map for the fingertip increased in size during training; however, the skin surface area represented by each nerve cell in the brain map became smaller, leading to greater refinement in performing the task. W. M. Jenkins, M. M. Merzenich, M. T. Ochs, T. Allard, and E. Guic-Robles, 1990, "Functional Reorganization of Primary Somatosensory Cortex in Adult Owl Monkeys After Behaviorally Controlled Tactile Stimulation," *Journal of Neurophysiology* 63(1):82–104.

      Subsequent experiments extended similar findings to the motor cortex. Since acquisition and execution of a skilled motor task require the coordinated participation of a number of brain structures, including the motor cortex, the basal ganglia, the cerebellum, and the spinal cord, the experimenters find it reasonable to assume that such differentiation through experience is widespread throughout the brain. R. J. Nudo, G. W. Milliken, W. M. Jenkins, and M. M. Merzenich. 1996, "Use-Dependent Alterations of Movement Representations in Primary Motor Cortex of Adult Squirrel Monkeys," *Journal of Neuroscience* 16(2):785–807.

254   While differentiation is most active in the first few years following birth: During the "critical period" of early development, a child is able to attend and remember what they are experiencing, allowing effortless differentiation of brain maps. In adulthood, such differentiation is possible but requires training our focused attention and awareness. M. P. Kilgard and M. M. Merzenich, 1998, "Cortical Map Reorganization Enabled by Nucleus Basalis Activity," *Science* 279(5357):1714–1718.

255   "improvement or refinement through increased complexity": One neuroscientist whose view of a possible mechanism of consciousness truly embraces the notion of complexity is Gerald Edelman. He concludes that high values of complexity correspond to an optimal blend of functional specialization (or differentiation) and functional integration within a system. "This is clearly the case for systems like the brain—different areas and groups of neurons do different things (they are differentiated) at the same time they interact to give rise to a unified conscious scene and to unified behaviors (they are integrated). By contrast, systems whose individual elements are either not integrated (such as a gas) or not specialized (like a homogenous crystal) will have minimal complexity." For Edelman, consciousness is a continuously shifting association of groups of neurons showing an overall coherent behavior but able to group and regroup dynamically according to their specific functional interactions. In other words, it is complex. A deteriorating brain has many groups, but they are poorly associated (compare the gas, above). By contrast, brain activity is highly synchronized in epilepsy or slow-wave sleep, showing integration and order but little specialization (compare the crystal). Neither of these dysfunctional states demonstrate complexity. G. M. Edelman and G. Tononi, 2000, *A Universe of Consciousness: How Matter Becomes Imagination* (New York: Basic Books), 130–133.

255   *the impossible possible, the possible comfortable, and the comfortable elegant:* One of the most quoted of the sayings of Dr. Moshe Feldenkrais in demonstrating the process underlying human progress.

258   Research shows that hours of solving crossword puzzles, travel-
       ing to new places, or doing rote exercises do not necessarily in-
       crease differentiation: Researchers at Georgia Tech found no
       evidence that crossword-puzzle solving reduced, in older adults,
       the known age-related decline in problem-solving ability. They
       mostly rely on general knowledge. D. Z. Hambrick, T. A. Salt-
       house, and E. J. Meinz, 1999, "Predictors of Crossword Puzzle
       Proficiency and Moderators of Age-cognition Relations," *Journal
       of Experimental Psychology: General* 128(2):131–164.

       By applying elements of the Nine Essentials, however, any pas-
       times can be transformed into a supremely beneficial activity for
       promoting vitality, and a number of researchers are publishing
       more-positive results in studies that look at programs designed
       specifically to address brain plasticity. H. W. Mahncke, B. B. Con-
       nor, J. Appelman, O. N. Ahsanuddin, J. L. Hardy, R. A. Wood, N.
       M. Joyce, T. Boniske, S. M. Atkins, and M. M. Merzenich, 2006,
       "Memory Enhancement in Healthy Older Adults Using a Brain
       Plasticity–Based Training Program: A Randomized, Controlled
       Study," *PNAS* 103(33):12523–12528.

       Lawrence C. Katz, Ph.D., a professor of neurobiology at Duke
       University, says such exercises help the brain to not only maintain
       connections between nerve cells—and thus preserve memory re-
       call—but also aid in developing new connections. The mental de-
       cline most people experience is due to the atrophy of connections
       between nerve cells in the brain as a result of routine behaviors.
       J. Volz, 2000, "Successful Aging: The Second 50; Psychologists'
       Research Is Changing Attitudes About What It Takes to Live
       the Good—and Longer—Life," *Monitor on Psychology* 31(1).
       http://www.apa.org/monitor/jan00/cs.html.

Bibliography

Amen, D. 2005. *Making a Good Brain Great*. New York: Harmony Books.

Bannister, R. 2004. *The Four-Minute Mile*. Revised and enlarged edition. Lyons Press.

Begley, S. 2007. *Train Your Mind, Change Your Brain*. New York: Ballantine Books.

Bergson, H. 1998. *Creative Evolution*. New York: Dover.

Bernstein, N. A. 1996. *On Dexterity and Its Development*. Translated by M. L. Latash. Mahwah, N.J.: Lawrence Erlbaum.

Berthoz, A. 2000. *The Brain's Sense of Movement*. Translated by Giselle Weiss. Cambridge, Mass.: Harvard University Press.

Brown, M., and A. O'Connor. 1985. *Woman Talk*. London: Futura Publications.

Csikszentmihalyi, M. 1990. *Flow: The Psychology of Optimal Experience*. New York: Harper Perennial.

Damasio, A. R. 1994. *Descartes' Error: Emotion, Reason and the Human Brain*. New York: Grosset/Putnam.

———. 1999. *The Feeling of What Happens: Body and Emotion in the Making of Consciousness*. London: William Heinemann.

Dennett, D. C. 1991. *Consciousness Explained*. Boston: Little, Brown.

Doidge, N. 2007. *The Brain That Changes Itself*. New York: Viking Penguin.

Edelman, G. M. 1992. *Bright Air, Brilliant Fire: On the Matter of the Mind*. New York: Basic Books.

———. 2005. *Wider Than the Sky*. New Haven, Conn.: Yale University Press.

Edelman, G. M., and G. Tononi. 2000. *A Universe of Consciousness: How Matter Becomes Imagination*. New York: Basic Books.

Eliot, L. 1999. *What's Going On in There? How the Brain and Mind Develop in the First Five Years of Life*. New York: Bantam.

Feldenkrais, M. 1990. *Awareness Through Movement*. New York: Harper-Collins.

Freud, S. 2005. *Civilization and Its Discontents*. New York: W. W. Norton.

Gladwell, M. 2000. *The Tipping Point: How Little Things Can Make a Big Difference*. Boston: Little, Brown.

Gopnik, A., A. N. Meltzoff, P. K. Kuhl. 1999. *The Scientist in the Crib: Minds, Brains, and How Children Learn*. New York: William Morrow.

Gould, S. J. 2007. *Ever Since Darwin*. New York: W. W. Norton.

Guyton, A. C. 1981. *Textbook of Medical Physiology*. Philadelphia: Saunders.

Hayward, J. W., and F. J. Varela, eds. 2001. *Gentle Bridges: Conversations with the Dalai Lama on the Sciences of Mind*. Boston: Shambhala.

Hebb, D. O. 1949. *The Organization of Behaviour*. New York: Wiley.

Huxley, L. Archera. 1995. *You Are Not the Target*. Portland, OR: Metamorphous Press.

Jaffe, D., and C. Scott. 1988. *Take This Job and Love It*. New York: Fireside.

Kandel, E. R. 2007. *In Search of Memory: The Emergence of a New Science of Mind*. New York: W. W. Norton.

Klein, M. 2002. *Beyond Orgasm*. San Francisco: Celestial Arts.

Koch, C. 2004. *The Quest for Consciousness: A Neurobiological Approach*. Roberts, Englewood, Colo.: Roberts and Company Publishers.

LeDoux, J. 2002. *Synaptic Self: How Our Brains Become Who We Are*. New York: Viking Penguin.

Lehninger, A. 1993. *Principles of Biochemistry*, 2nd ed. New York: Worth.

Llinàs, R., and P. S. Churchland, eds. 1996. *The Mind-Brain Continuum*. Boston: MIT Press.

Maslov, A. 1971. *The Farther Reaches of Human Nature*. New York: Viking Press.

———. 1998. *Toward a Psychology of Being*. 3rd ed. New York: Wiley.

Milne, A. A. 1926. *Winnie-the-Pooh*. London: Methuen.

Norretranders, T. 1998. *The User Illusion: Cutting Consciousness Down to Size*. New York: Viking Penguin.

Pagels, H. 1989. *The Dreams of Reason: The Computer and the Rise of the Sciences of Complexity*. New York: Bantam Books.

Patmore, A. 2006. *The Truth About Stress*. London: Atlantic Books.

Prasad, K. N. 1980. *Regulation of Differentiation in Mammalian Nerve Cells*. New York: Plenum.

Ramachandran, V. S. 2003. *The Emerging Mind. The Reith Lectures, 2003*. London: Profile Books.

Ratey, J. J. 2000. *A User's Guide to the Brain*. New York: Pantheon.

Roberts, G. C. 1992. *Motivation in Sport and Exercise*. Champaign, IL: Human Kinetics.

Schwartz, J. M., and S. Begley. 2003. *The Mind and the Brain: Neuroplasticity and the Power of Mental Force*. New York: ReganBooks.

Stapp, H. P. 2007. *Mindful Universe: Quantum Mechanics and the Participating Observer*. Berlin: Springer-Verlag.

Thelen, E., and L. B. Smith. 1994. *A Dynamic Systems Approach to the Development of Cognition and Action*. Cambridge, Mass.: MIT Press.

Thompson, D. 1961. *On Growth and Form*. Canto ed. Cambridge: Cambridge University Press.

Tolle, E. 1999. *The Power of Now*. Novato, California: New World Library.

Westney, W. 2006. *The Perfect Wrong Note: Learning to Trust Your Musical Self*. Pompton Plains, N.J.: Amadeus Press.

Acknowledgments

I'M DEEPLY GRATEFUL to all my clients for the opportunity to be part of the process of transforming their lives for the better. I am especially indebted to all the parents who brought their children with special needs to me, willing to take the less traveled, *alternative* route. It is through these tens of thousands of interactions that NeuroMovement for lifelong vitality was conceptualized.

I have been blessed with an incredible co-writer, Hal Zina Bennett. During the process, Hal was a lot more than just a fabulous writer. His wisdom, curiosity, warmth, integrity, and remarkable knowledge and experience have enriched and deepened every page of this book.

I'm deeply grateful to David Gerstein for keeping his promise to draw the illustrations in the midst of his very busy and demanding life. His amazing talent, generosity, and friendship move me, and I'm honored to have his work be a part of this book.

I can't thank Neil Sharp, M.D., enough for the countless hours he has put into exploring brain plasticity research and the many illuminating discussions we have had on the topic.

My editor, Julia Pastore, "got it" right away, realizing the newness in the thinking and the relevance and importance of the Nine Essentials to people's lives. Her comments and suggestions always helped clarify and elevate the book. Shaye Areheart, Kira Walton, Melanie DeNardo, Cindy Berman, and the rest of the team at Harmony Books were always right there, enthusiastically doing their incredible work.

I'm very grateful to my agent, Matthew Carnicelli, at Carnicelli Literary Management, for his intellectual curiosity, his understanding of the materials, his dedication, and for guiding me so skillfully through the process.

I want to thank my colleague and friend Marcy Lindheimer for always seeing me with such good eyes and having endless trust in my abilities. I am deeply grateful to Randy Methven for her friendship and her inspired, fierce coaching, never letting me off the hook. I feel so lucky to share with my childhood friend, Dr. Eilat Almagor, a parallel professional path. Thank you for your brilliance, humor, and the many illuminating conversations about the brain, movement, research, and much more. I thank Joseph Feinstein for always being there to help in any way possible.

My gratitude goes to Robert Blumenfeld for his patience, love, and support of me and my work during the writing of this book, and to my daughter, Sacha Baniel-Stark, who is a constant manifestation of brain plasticity and endless possibilities, and for making it okay that her mom focused on her work so much of the time.

My thanks to Liza and Raz Ingraci, Betsy Sanders, Karen Leland, and Asia Swartz for their friendship and support throughout the process, and to my dear friend Marianne Kagan, who has since passed away, for years of encouragement. I thank my brother, Eran Baniel, for his patience and understanding, waiting for me to take some time away from writing this book while we were developing the Desk-Trainer Program. My gratitude to Gerald Sindel for helping me, in the early stages, think through, clarify, and hone in on the Nine Essentials.

I thank my co-teachers in the Anat Baniel Method, my clients, and my students for nudging me to write this book, and for their interest, enthusiasm, and feedback.

This book and the work it is based upon would not be possible without the many outstanding teachers I have had the good fortune to learn from. To mention just a few: Moshe Feldenkrais transformed my life in ways I could have never known to ask for and gave me the tools and understanding from which to develop my own methods of working with others. Amos Tversky taught me ways to bring mathematical thinking into the study and understanding of human behavior and made it fun! My father, Avram Baniel, a scientist, instilled in me the love for thinking and knowledge and was the one to sign me up for Archipova Grossman's dance class, where, at age seven, I realized for the first time the power of awareness to transform body, mind, and heart. Dr. Larry Epstein trusted in my knowledge and encouraged me to put it in writing. His insights helped guide the way. Itamar Rogovsky's training of clinical psychologists in a program attempting to prevent PTSD in combat soldiers taught me the importance of real outcomes in real life. The Hoffman Process teachers demonstrated how love is an action and can be taught.

Finally, I would like to express my immense gratitude to the many neuroscientists who dedicate their time and brilliance to researching and bringing greater understanding to this most incredible, fascinating, and challenging topic—the human brain. The discoveries and theories of Michael Merzenich, Nancy Byl, Alvaro Pascual-Leone, Richard Davidson, Fred Gage, Richard Passingham, Eric Kandel, and Vilayanur Ramachandran, to mention just a few, are opening new possibilities for all of us to live better, healthier, more satisfying lives. We are all lucky to have so many wonderful books that make this emerging knowledge available to all of us. Sharon Begley, Daniel Amen, Jeffery Schwartz, Norman Doidge, Gerald Adelman, Mark Latsh, Antonio Damasio, and Dharma Singh Khalsa are just some of the authors who deserve our recognition and appreciation for their great work.

Index

Academic learning, 60
Action steps for enthusiasm,
    165–166
Amen, Daniel G., 58, 59
Anat Baniel Method Center, San
    Rafael, California, 11
Animals Are Beautiful People
    (documentary film), 183–185
Archimedes, 64, 65
Aristotle, 48
Armstrong, Louis. 46
Ascent of Man, The (Bronowski),
    251
Attention
    differed from awareness, 235
    to movement (*see* Movement with
        Attention)
    power of, 40–42
Auditory learning, 59–60
Automatic movement, 34–35, 37, 38
Automatic response, 237–238
Awareness, 20, 234–252, 253, 261
    as action, 243–244
    benefits of, 236–237
    defined. 235
    differed from attention, 235
    examples, 238–239, 249–251
    exercises, 240–241, 244–248, 252
    observation and, 241–243
    vitality quotient exercise, 252

Baboons, 184–185, 188, 197
Bach-y-Rita, Paul, 84
Background effort, 96–97
Bannister, Roger, 74
Bateson, Patrick, 189
Beginner's mind, 56–58
Begley, Sharon, 173
Being in the now, 81, 94
Bernstein, Nicholai A., 110–111
Beyond Orgasm (Klein), 220
Blame, as learning switch turnoff,
    72, 73
Boredom, 52
Brain Workouts, 58, 59
Bronowski, Jacob, 251
Buddhist teachings, 56
Burnout, 43

Campbell, Joseph, 206, 224
Canfield, Jack, 223, 224, 231
Cantor, Eddie, 134
Carroll, Lewis, 9–10
Chicken Soup for the Soul
    (Canfield), 223
Childhood
    development, 7, 30–31
    emotions in, 99
    excitement in, 166–167
    self-discovery in, 190–191,
        195–196

Childhood *(cont'd)*
  skill mastery in, 145
  variation and, 117
Civilization and Its Discontents
  (Freud), 70
Common sense, 173
Communication, variation and,
  119
Crum, Alia J., 217
Csikszentmihalyi, Mihaly, 140
Curiosity, 78

Dalai Lama, 234
Davidson, Richard, 157
Daydreaming, 207–210, 221
Defensiveness, 72
Diamond, Marian, 58–59
Differentiation, process of, 254–256,
  258
Doctor Zhivago (Pasternak), 224
Dreams (*see* Imagination and
  Dreams)

eBay, 203
Eeyorism, 172–173
Einstein, Albert, vii, 23, 58, 77, 154,
  173, 206, 225, 233
Elegance, 82–84
Ellis, Havelock, 182
Emotion as movement, 39–40
Emotional intensity, reducing, 90–91
Emotional life, subtlety in, 99–102
Endorphins, 35
Enthusiasm, 19, 156–181, 253, 261
  action steps for, 165–166, 180
  examples, 157–161, 169–171,
    174–175, 178–180
  from excitement to, 166–168
  exercises, 161–164, 168–169,
    175–176, 178, 181
  and free choice, 176–178
  generosity and, 178
  lack of, 171–173
  origin of word, 178
  reclaiming power of, 169–171

as skill, 157–161
  vitality quotient exercise, 181
Entropy, 177
Ever Since Darwin (Gould), 188, 204
Examples of Nine Essentials for
  Vitality
  Awareness, 238–239, 249–251
  Enthusiasm, 157–161, 169–171,
    174–175, 178–180
  Flexible Goals, 185–186, 200–201
  Imagination and Dreams,
    215–217, 222–223, 226–230
  Learning Switch, 53–56, 62–64
  Movement with Attention, 31–33,
    35–37, 44–46
  Slow, 136–137, 142–143,
    145–146, 152–153
  Subtlety, 93–98, 100–101
  Variation, 109–110, 112–114,
    121–126
Excessive force, use of, 83, 89–90,
  94–95, 97–98, 100, 102
Excitement to enthusiasm, 166–168
Exercises (*see also* Vitality quotient)
  attentive hand, 40–41
  awareness, 240–241, 244–248
  beginner's mind, 56–58
  boosting intelligence, 103
  coming to life through enthusiasm,
    161–164
  comparing present with past,
    52–53
  daydreaming, 210
  dream action plan, 231
  dream board, 223–224
  experience new freedom of move-
    ment, 65–69
  feeling hand, 138–139
  flexible goals, 191–195, 202–203
  generating enthusiasm, 168–169
  generosity and enthusiasm, 178
  imagination, 212–214, 218–219
  leadership as path to vitality,
    175–176
  learning switch turnoffs, 72–73

minimizing force, 84–88
movement of emotions, 39–40
moving while thinking, 33–34
reading upside down, 108–109
reducing emotional intensity,
90–91
reducing force. 98
rigid goal setting, 187–188
slow listening, 141–142
small variations, big transformations, 118–119
take a slow break, 136
this leg is not that heavy, 147–150
touching toes, 114–117
transformational power of movement with attention, 26–30
use of variation to overcome pain,
127–129

Familiarity, in relationships, 139–140
Fangio, Juan, 104
Farther Reaches of Human Nature,
The (Maslow), 195
Fast, 134–136, 151–152
Fear
as Learning Switch turnoff, 73
Slow and, 142–145
Feldenkrais, Moshe, 1, 23, 60,
106–107, 200–201, 222–223,
225
Fight-or-flight response, 70
Fitzgerald, F. Scott, 196
Flexible Goals, 19–20, 182–205,
238, 253, 261
baboon case, 184–185, 188, 197
examples, 185–186, 200–201
exercises, 187–188, 191–195,
202–205
reversible approach, 196, 199,
201
rigid approach versus, 183–187,
195–197
steps for, 197–200
success and, 203–204
vitality quotient exercise, 204–205

Flow, 72
Flow: The Psychology of Optimal
Experience (Csikszentmihalyi),
140
Force
reducing, 82–84, 89–90, 95–98,
101
use of excessive, 83, 89–90,
94–95, 97–98, 100, 102
Free choice, enthusiasm and,
176–178
Freezing, 70–71
Freud, Sigmund, 70
Fuller, Buckminster, 253
Functional magnetic resonance
imaging (fMRI), 208

Gandhi, Mahatma, 234
Generosity, enthusiasm and, 178
Gentleness (see Subtlety)
Goals (see Flexible Goals)
Gould, Stephen Jay, 188, 204
Graham, Martha, 5
Gross, Ronald, 72
Guyton, Arthur C., 120

Habit (see Routine and habit)
Harvard Medical School, 17, 111
Hebb, Donald, 49
Hebbian plasticity, 49, 92, 151
Heroes, 81–82
Huxley, Aldous, 234
Huxley, Laura Archera, 138–139

"I Have a Dream. . . ." (King),
222
Imagination and Dreams, 13, 20,
206–233, 253, 261
daydreaming, 207–210, 221
discovering and following dreams,
224–225
examples. 215–217, 222–223,
226–230
exercises, 210, 212–214, 218–219,
223–224, 231–233

Imagination and Dreams *(cont'd)*
 harder to imagine than do,
  215–217
 power of dreams, 231–232
 power of imagination, 210–212,
  217–218
 steps for improving imagination,
  220–222
 vitality quotient exercise, 232–233
Inadequacy, feeling of, 72
Intellectual expression, 16
Intelligence, subtlety and, 102–103
Intentionality, 75–77
Intuition, subtlety and, 103–104
Iron, Ralph, 120

Jaffe, Dennis, 224
Joliot-Curie, Frédéric, 201

Kekulé, Friedrich, 120–121
Kelvin, Lord, 232
Kierkegaard, Søren, 106
Kinesthetic learning, 59–60
King, Martin Luther, Jr., 222, 224
Klein, Marty, 220
Knowledge, transformational power
  of, 10

Langer, Ellen J., 217
Lao-Tzu, 81
Leadership, as path to vitality,
  175–176
Leadership role, 78–79
Learning, types of, 59–65
Learning Switch, 18, 48–80, 253,
  260
 examples, 53–56, 62–64
 exercises, 52–53, 56–58, 65–69,
  72–73, 79–80
 turning on, 58–59, 72, 73–79
 turnoffs, 70–73
 types of learning, 59–65
 vitality quotient exercise, 79–80
Lee, Christopher, 204
L'Engle, Madeleine, 140

Levchin, Max, 203
Listening, slow, 141–142
Lynn, Stephen Jay, 208

Making a Good Brain Great
  (Amen), 58
Maslow, Abraham, 195, 225
Mason, Malia F., 208
Mead, Margaret, 139–140
Medawar, Peter, 76
Merzenich, Michael, 112, 176
Mistakes
 flexible goals and, 199, 202–203
 variation viewed as, 120–121,
  129–130
Mountain climbers, 81, 91
Movement with Attention, 18,
  23–47, 253, 260
 automatic movement versus,
  34–35, 37, 38
 emotion as movement, 39–40
 examples, 31–33, 35–37, 44–46
 exercises, 26–30, 33–34,
  39–41, 47
 movement, organization, and
  vitality, 30–34
 organization of movement,
  24–30, 46
 power of attention, 40–42
 routine and habit and, 42–44
 vitality quotient exercise, 47
Mozart, Wolfgang Amadeus, 190

National Aeronautics and Space
  Administration (NASA), 84
Negative entropy, 177, 228
Neurogenesis, 17
New York Times, 203, 232
Nine Essentials for Vitality, 16–17
 described, 18–20
 review of, 259–261
Now, being in the, 81, 94

Observation, awareness and,
  241–243

Ode magazine, 71
On Growth and Form (Thompson), 76
Oracle at Delphi, 234
Organic learning, 60, 61–64, 73–75, 78
Organization of movement, 24–30, 46

Pascual-Leone, Alvaro, 17, 111, 211
Past, comparing present with, 52–53
Past failures, as learning switch turnoff, 73
Pasternak, Boris, 224
Patmore, Angela, 71
PayPal, 203
Perlman, Itzhak, 257
Picasso, Pablo, 83
"Plastic Human Brain Cortex, The" (Pascual-Leone), 111
Play, 189, 198, 202
Power of Now, The (Tolle), 40, 81
Predictability, 51–52
Present, comparing with past, 52–53
Pruning process, 49
Psychological Science, 217

Racecar drivers, 81, 91
Reason, enthusiasm and, 173–175
Recombinant play, 77
REM (rapid eye movement) sleep, 209
Repetition, 107
Repetitive exercise, 38, 42, 113
Repression, 70
Reptilian brain, 70
Reversible approach, 196, 199, 201
Rhue, Judith, 208
Rigid approach, 183–187, 195–197
Rivlin, Gary, 203
Routine and habit, 17, 34–35, 37–38, 77
  breaking out of, 44
  seductiveness of, 42–43

Schumann, Clara, 156
Schwartz, Jeffrey, 173
Scott, Cynthia, 224
Self-affirmation, joy of, 196
Self-discovery, 190–191, 195–196
Self-knowledge, 234 (*see also* Awareness)
Self-trust, 72
Sensuality, Slow and, 137–140
Shichlul, 255, 257
Skill acquisition, 60–61
Skill mastery
  in childhood, 145
  Slow and, 145–146
Slow, 19, 134–155, 253, 261
  choices and, 152–153
  examples, 136–137, 142–143, 145–146, 152–153
  exercises, 136, 138–139, 141–142, 147–150, 154–155
  fast and, 134–136, 151–152
  negative connotations of, 134
  relationships and power of, 139–141
  sensuality and, 137–140
  skill mastery and, 145–146
  slow listening, 141–142
  stress and fear and, 142–145
  vitality quotient exercise, 154–155
Smithies, Oliver, 204
Socrates, 33
Stress, 71, 131–132, 142–145
Subtlety, 18–19, 81–105, 253, 260
  in emotional life, 99–102
  examples, 93–98, 100–101
  exercises, 84–88, 90–91, 98, 103, 105
  gain without strain, 94–96
  intelligence and, 102–103
  intuition and, 103–104
  minimize force to maximize attunement, 82–84
  perception of subtle differences, 91–94

Subtlety *(cont'd)*
    reducing force, 82–84, 89–90,
        95–98, 101
    use of excessive force, 83, 89–90,
        94–95, 97–98, 100, 102
    vitality quotient exercise, 105
Success, flexible goals and, 203–204
Survival responses, 176–177

Take This Job and Love It (Jaffe and
    Scott), 224
Textbook of Medical Physiology
    (Guyton), 120
Thinking, 102–103
Thompson, D'Arcy, 76–77
Thoreau, Henry David, 225
Through the Looking-Glass
    (Carroll), 9–10
To-do lists, 135, 136
Tolle, Eckhart, 40, 81, 91, 94
*Train Your Mind, Change Your
    Brain* (Begley), 173
Truth About Stress, The (Patmore),
    71

Unamuno, Miguel de, 131

Variation, 19, 106–133, 238, 253,
    261
    communication and, 119
    creating, 131
    as essential, 117–118
    examples, 109–110, 112–114,
        121–126
    excluding, 111–112
    exercises, 108–109, 114–119,
        127–129, 132–133
    extreme case of deprivation of,
        121–122

moving forward with, 113–114
    pain and, 124–129
    stress and, 131–132
    viewed as mistake, 120–121,
        129–130
    vitality quotient exercise,
        132–133
Visual learning, 59
Vitality (*see* Awareness; Enthusiasm;
    Flexible Goals; Imagination and
    Dreams; Learning Switch;
    Movement with Attention;
    Slow; Subtlety; Variation)
Vitality quotient
    Awareness, 252
    Enthusiasm, 181
    Flexible Goals, 204–205
    Imagination and Dreams,
        232–233
    Learning Switch, 79–80
    Movement with Attention, 47
    Slow, 154–155
    Subtlety, 105
    Variation, 132–133

Warrior mentality, 82
Washington Post, 204
Weber, Ernst Heinrich, 96
Westney, William, 130
Wilson, Matthew, 209–210
Winnie-the-Pooh (Milne), 172
Wright brothers, 232

Yemen, 107
Yoga, variation in, 119
You Are Not the Target (Huxley),
    138–139

Zukav, Gary, 225

About Anat Baniel

Born and raised in Israel, Anat is the author of two highly acclaimed books: *Move Into Life: The Nine Essentials for Lifelong Vitality* (a San Francisco Chronicle bestseller), and *Kids Beyond Limits: The Anat Baniel Method for Awakening the Brain and Transforming the Life of Your Special Needs Child,* as well as numerous videos on NeuroMovement®. She is the originator of The Anat Baniel Method® and NeuroMovement®.

As a world renowned teacher and trainer, Anat has been called a "miracle worker" for her ability to bring new life and vitality to tens of thousands of people of all ages and conditions: healthy young adults pursuing peak performance in sports and other endeavors; those experiencing common aches and limitations; and people in their advanced years seeking greater vitality. She has helped infants and small children with developmental difficulties to achieve goals previously thought impossible by their medical professionals.

Thirty years ago the unparalleled outcomes produced by her highly innovative work challenged what was then the scientific consensus that the brain could not change itself beyond the very early years of life. Today her distinctive methods are endorsed by leading brain scientists, medical doctors, and others in the helping professions, and are supported by cutting edge scientific discoveries in *neuroplasticity*—the brain's ability to change and regenerate itself throughout life.

To date Anat has trained hundreds of Anat Baniel Method practitioners who help adults and children suffering stroke and brain injury, aches, pains, and other limiting factors, to attain new levels of performance and well-being. Her work redefines what it means to be fit, awake, and alive.

Anat and her team of trainers offer practitioner training programs. In addition, Anat teaches workshops and makes presentations worldwide, including France, England, Japan, Sweden, Germany, and Israel.

Anat was recently invited to conduct research and participate in a project aimed at transforming traditional rehabilitation into a neuroscience/neuroplasticity-based rehabilitation process.

Visit her website at www.AnatBanielMethod.com.

If you enjoyed reading this book and would like to further enhance your vitality, I have a gift I would like to share with you. Please go to my website, WWW.ANATBANIELMETHOD.COM, and download your *"Move into Life* Free Class" with me.

ANAT BANIEL METHOD CENTER
in San Rafael, California

THE ANAT BANIEL METHOD CENTER moved to its new head-quarters in 2005. Practitioners in the Center offer private sessions to adults seeking to improve their physical and mental performance and overcome pain and limitation due to accidents, illness, and lifelong injurious habits, and to babies and children with special needs ranging from brain damage and genetic disorders to learning disabilities. Practitioner certification training programs, weekend workshops, free presentations, and weekly classes are offered on a regular basis.

Additional Anat Baniel Method Centers are located in:

Anat Baniel Center of San Jose, California
Contact: andreabowers@abmcentersanjose.com

The Children's Practice: The Anat Baniel Method for Children, New York, New York
Contact: mlindheimr@aol.com

Visit our website at AnatBanielMethod.com:

- Find an Anat Baniel Method Center and practitioners near you
- Try free online movement lessons
- Watch Anat work with special-needs children
- Sign up for our online animated movement coach (www.desk-trainer.com)
- Register for a weekend seminar
- Become a practitioner (www.anatbanieltraining.com)
- Hear the true stories of our successes (and challenges), and share your experience
- Purchase DVD and CD movement programs to heal healthy backs, necks, and joints; increase vitality; and approach working with special-needs children

Made in the USA
Las Vegas, NV
08 June 2023

73124192R00184